# HOW
# TO GET
# THE DRAGONS
# OUT OF
# YOUR
# TEMPLE

# HOW TO GET THE DRAGONS OUT OF YOUR TEMPLE

### DIANE NEUMAN

## CELESTIAL ARTS
## MILLBRAE CALIFORNIA

First printing:  February, 1976
Manufactured in the United States of America

**Library of Congress Cataloging in Publication Data**

Neuman, Diane.
    How to get the dragons out of your temple.

    1.  Yoga, hatha.    I.  Title.
R.A.781.7.N48      613.7      75-28760
ISBN 0-89087-118-3

1 2 3 4 5 6 7 8 9 – 80 79 78 77 76

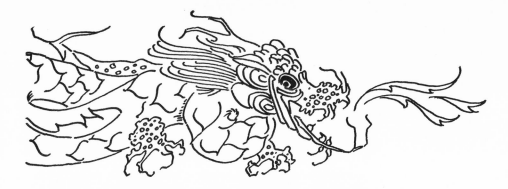

# CONTENTS

# INTRODUCTION

YOUR BODY IS TRULY THE TEMPLE
OF YOUR MIND AND SPIRIT....
WITHIN THIS TEMPLE, YOU MUST
LIVE, LEARN, TEACH, DREAM,
LOVE, AND HOPEFULLY
STRIVE TO REACH YOUR
FULL POTENTIAL AS A
HUMAN BEING!

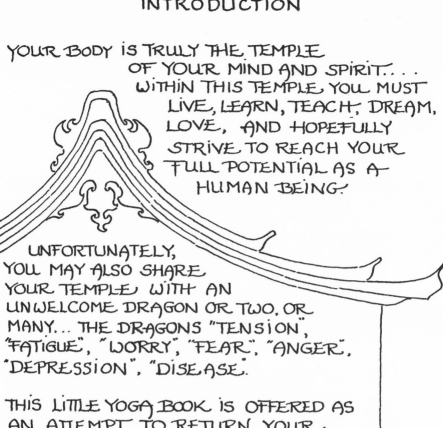

UNFORTUNATELY,
YOU MAY ALSO SHARE
YOUR TEMPLE WITH AN
UNWELCOME DRAGON OR TWO, OR
MANY... THE DRAGONS "TENSION",
"FATIGUE", "WORRY", "FEAR", "ANGER",
"DEPRESSION", "DISEASE".

THIS LITTLE YOGA BOOK IS OFFERED AS
AN ATTEMPT TO RETURN YOUR
TEMPLE TO YOU, THE RIGHTFUL
OWNER.

MAY YOUR TEMPLE
ALWAYS BE FREE
OF

DRAGONS.

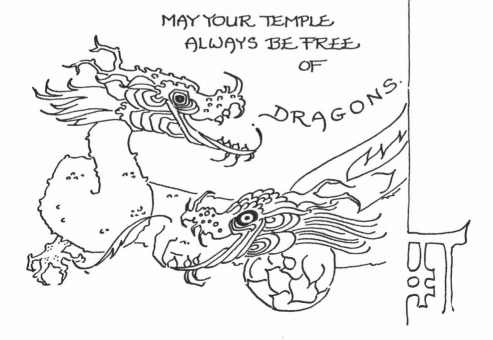

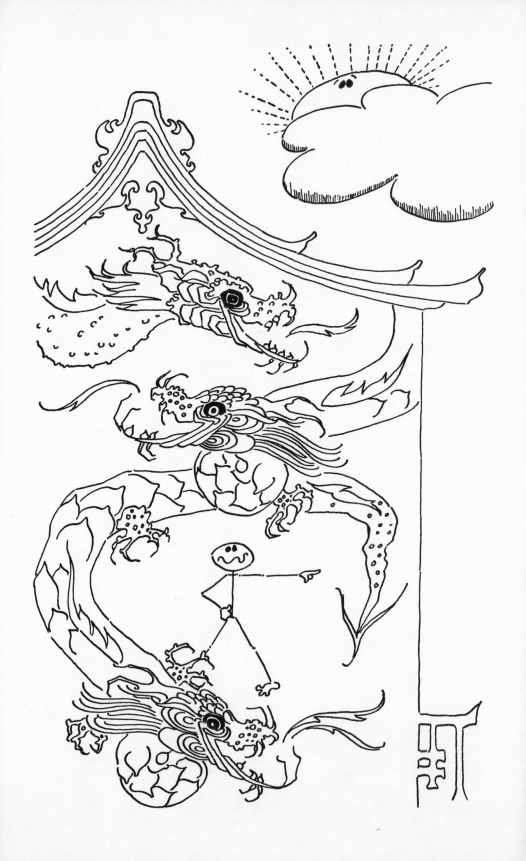

YOGA

is a sanskrit
word meaning
yoke or union...
the joining of
a healthy body
and disciplined
mind for the
purpose of
spiritual
growth.

YOGA

is growing,
unfolding
.... . becoming.

# ASANA

AN ASANA IS AN ANCIENT YOGIC POSE, POSTURE, OR EXERCISE — A POSE THAT PROVIDES THE OPPORTUNITY TO COORDINATE YOUR MIND, BODY, AND SPIRIT.... THE HARMONY THAT IS BORN WITH THE PRACTICE OF THE POSES WILL RADIATE AND ENRICH EVERY MOMENT OF YOUR DAILY LIFE.... REGULAR PRACTICE OF THE ASANAS WILL ENABLE YOU TO DISCIPLINE, REFINE, PROTECT EVERY MUSCLE, NERVE, AND GLAND.... THE ASANAS ARE MEDITATION IN MOTION.

# PRANAYAMA

PRANAYAMA IS THE SEARCH FOR, THE STORING OF, THE WISE SPENDING OF VITAL ENERGY BY STUDYING AND CONTROLLING THE BREATH..... YOUR BREATH IS A PRECIOUS AND POWERFUL GIFT FROM NATURE .... A MAGIC GENIE AWAITING YOUR INSTRUCTIONS...

YOUR GENIE —
OFFERS YOU ENDURANCE AND VITALITY,
CARRIES YOU INTO THE SUBTLE DEPTHS
                    OF YOUR MIND,
SHIELDS YOU FROM INFECTION,
SHEPHERDS YOUR EMOTIONS,
QUIETS YOUR FEARS,
BRINGS YOU PEACE AND REST.

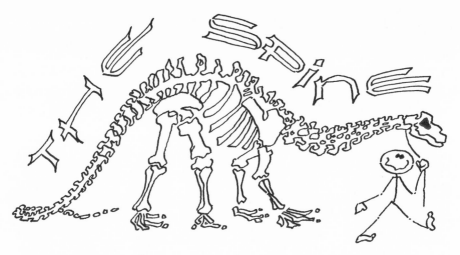

YOUR SPINE IS THE AXIS OF YOUR BODY. THIS STRONG FLEXIBLE TOWER OF BONES IS AN ENGINEERING WONDER THAT WILL WORK WELL FOR YOU, IF YOU UNDERSTAND AND PROTECT IT. THE SPINE IS A STACK OF BONY KNOBBY SPOOLS (VERTEBRAE) ARRANGED IN A GENTLE "S" SHAPE. THE VERTEBRAE ARE HELD APART BY SPONGY PLATES (DISCS) THAT PREVENT WEAR AND FRICTION AS YOU MOVE. AS YOU WALK, THE SHOCK OF YOUR STEP IS ABSORBED BY: THE ARCH IN YOUR FOOT, THE DISCS BETWEEN YOUR VERTEBRAE, AND THE NATURAL SPRING OF THE SPINE'S "S"-SHAPE. THUS, YOUR BRAIN IS SPARED THE JARRING DESTRUCTIVE SHOCK THAT WOULD OTHERWISE TRAVEL UP YOUR BODY TO YOUR HEAD WITH EACH STEP.

YOUR SPINE GUARDS AND CHANNELS THE DELICATE, COMPLEX NETWORK OF NERVES WHICH DESCENDS FROM THE BRAIN TO ALL PARTS OF THE BODY.

THE VERTEBRAE SERVE AS ANCHORS FOR A SERIES OF ATTACHED MUSCLES, LIGAMENTS, AND TENDONS.

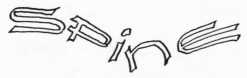

**SPINE**

7 SMALL DELICATE VERTEBRAE FORM THE CERVICAL CURVE AT THE BACK OF THE NECK.

12 THORACIC VERTEBRAE FORM THE OUT-CURVE OF YOUR UPPER BACK AND ARE THE SOURCE OF YOUR 12 PAIRS OF RIBS

5 HEAVY LUMBAR VERTEBRAE FORM THE IN-CURVE AT THE BACK OF YOUR WAIST

BENEATH THE LUMBAR IS THE SACRUM, A FLAT TRIANGULAR BONY FORMATION MADE UP OF 5 SEPARATE VERTEBRAE THAT FUSE INTO 1 FORMATION IN ADULTS

AT THE LOWER END OF THE SPINE IS THE COCCYX, A "TAIL" OF 4 TINY BONES

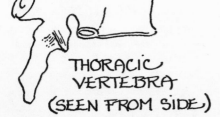

THORACIC VERTEBRA (SEEN FROM SIDE)

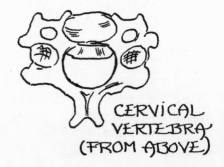

CERVICAL VERTEBRA (FROM ABOVE)

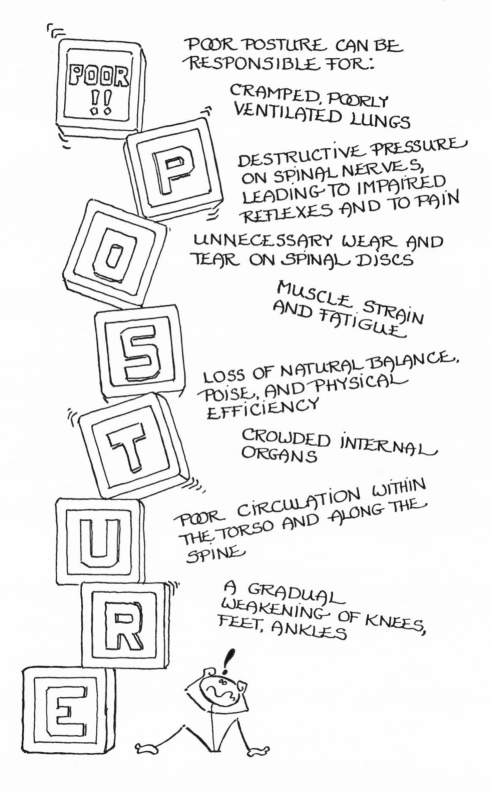

POOR POSTURE CAN BE
RESPONSIBLE FOR:

CRAMPED, POORLY
VENTILATED LUNGS

DESTRUCTIVE PRESSURE
ON SPINAL NERVES,
LEADING TO IMPAIRED
REFLEXES AND TO PAIN

UNNECESSARY WEAR AND
TEAR ON SPINAL DISCS

MUSCLE STRAIN
AND FATIGUE

LOSS OF NATURAL BALANCE,
POISE, AND PHYSICAL
EFFICIENCY

CROWDED INTERNAL
ORGANS

POOR CIRCULATION WITHIN
THE TORSO AND ALONG THE
SPINE

A GRADUAL
WEAKENING OF KNEES,
FEET, ANKLES

## CARE OF THE SPINE

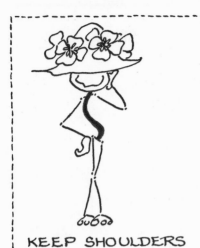

KEEP SHOULDERS
AND HIPS LEVEL

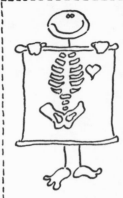

HAVE
REGULAR
MEDICAL
CHECK-UPS

GET
PLENTY OF
REST

EAT A
WELL-
BALANCED
DIET

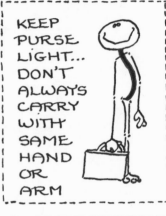

KEEP
PURSE
LIGHT...
DON'T
ALWAYS
CARRY
WITH
SAME
HAND
OR
ARM

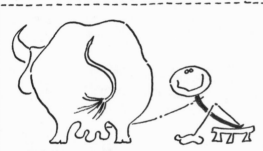

PLACE OFFICE AND
KITCHEN EQUIPMENT
WITHIN EASY REACH

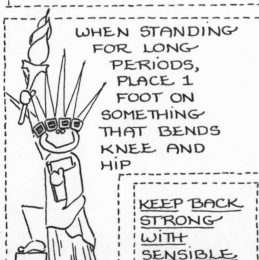

WHEN STANDING
FOR LONG
PERIODS,
PLACE 1
FOOT ON
SOMETHING
THAT BENDS
KNEE AND
HIP

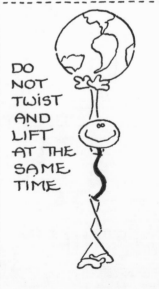

DO
NOT
TWIST
AND
LIFT
AT THE
SAME
TIME

KEEP BACK
STRONG
WITH
SENSIBLE
DAILY
EXERCISE

## CARE OF THE SPINE

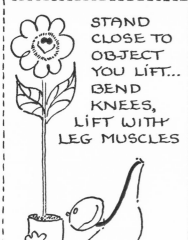

STAND CLOSE TO OBJECT YOU LIFT... BEND KNEES, LIFT WITH LEG MUSCLES

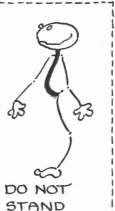

DO NOT STAND WITH KNEES LOCKED BACK

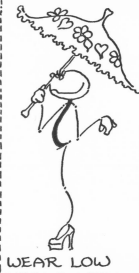

WEAR LOW HEELS, WELL-FIT SHOES

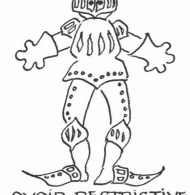

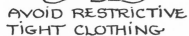

AVOID RESTRICTIVE TIGHT CLOTHING

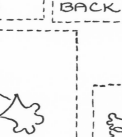
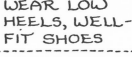

SLEEP ON YOUR SIDE...MATTRESS SHOULD ALLOW SPINE TO REST IN A STRAIGHT LINE

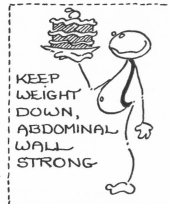

KEEP WEIGHT DOWN, ABDOMINAL WALL STRONG

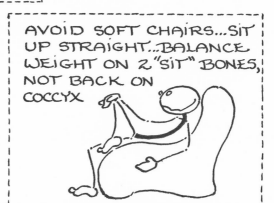

AVOID SOFT CHAIRS...SIT UP STRAIGHT...BALANCE WEIGHT ON 2 "SIT" BONES, NOT BACK ON COCCYX

WE WERE ORIGINALLY DESIGNED TO WALK ON 4, NOT 2, LEGS. ALTHOUGH WE ARE ADAPTING SLOWLY TO THE RADICAL CHANGE IN BODY POSITION, THE CHANGE IS FAR FROM COMPLETE.. ...

THE UPRIGHT POSTURE LIFTED OUR SENSING EQUIPMENT UP TO A MORE FAVORABLE LEVEL. OUR HANDS WERE FREED. HOWEVER, OUR NEW POSTURE CAUSES OUR SINUS CAVITIES TO DRAIN POORLY. NOW THE SENSITIVE LUMBAR SPINE MUST BEAR THE WEIGHT OF THE ENTIRE UPPER BODY. THE VISCERAL ORGANS OF THE ABDOMEN, INSTEAD OF HANGING FREE, ARE PILED ONE ON TOP OF THE OTHER. THE THE MUSCULAR SHEATH COVERING THE ABDOMEN, WHICH WAS ONCE CREATED AS A SIMPLE FLOOR, MUST NOW SERVE AS A RETAINING WALL. THE HEART HAS THE ADDITIONAL WORK OF PULLING BLOOD FROM THE FEET, STRAIGHT UP TO THE BRAIN AND VITAL GLANDS OF THE UPPER BODY.

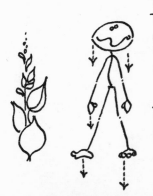

IT IS, THEREFORE, NECESSARY TO KEEP THE SUPPORT MUSCLES OF THE SPINE AND THE ABDOMEN VERY STRONG. THE BODY MUST BE REGULARLY INVERTED TO REVERSE THE DESTRUCTIVE EFFECTS OF GRAVITY'S CONSTANT DOWNWARD PULL ON THE BODY.

ABOUT 2/3 OF YOUR BODY WEIGHT IS WATER. EACH CELL IS A TINY FLOATING MARINE ORGANISM.

WATER IS VITAL IN REGULATING YOUR BODY TEMPERATURE. WATER ACTS AS CARRIER FOR THE BLOOD...

WATER IS IMPORTANT IN ALL THE BODY'S BUILDING WORK..

WATER IS ESSENTIAL FOR CLEARING THE BODY OF WASTE....

WATER ACTS TO MAINTAIN INTERNAL CLEANLINESS AND VITALITY IN YOUR ENTIRE BODY......

EVERY DAY YOU LOSE ABOUT 3 PINTS OF FLUID FROM YOUR KIDNEYS....

AND YOU LOSE ABOUT 1½ TO 2 PINTS OF FLUID THROUGH YOUR SKIN .....

10-15 OUNCES ARE LOST BY WAY OF YOUR LUNGS...

AND A LITTLE BIT MORE VIA TEARS, BOWELS. ETC. ...

THAT'S OVER 5 PINTS IN 24 HOURS...

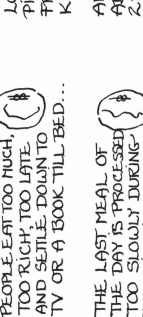
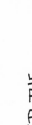
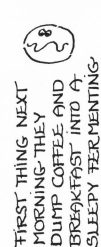

MOST SEDENTARY PEOPLE EAT TOO MUCH, TOO RICH, TOO LATE AND SETTLE DOWN TO TV OR A BOOK TILL BED...

THE LAST MEAL OF THE DAY IS PROCESSED TOO SLOWLY DURING THE NIGHT....

AS THEY SLEEP, THE LUNGS AND SINUS CAVITIES DRAIN INTO THE STOMACH.....

FIRST THING NEXT MORNING-THEY DUMP COFFEE AND BREAKFAST INTO A SLEEPY FERMENTING STOMACH....

INSTEAD, SIP A SMALL GLASS OF HOT WATER. PUT BREAKFAST INTO A CLEAN, AWAKE SYSTEM!

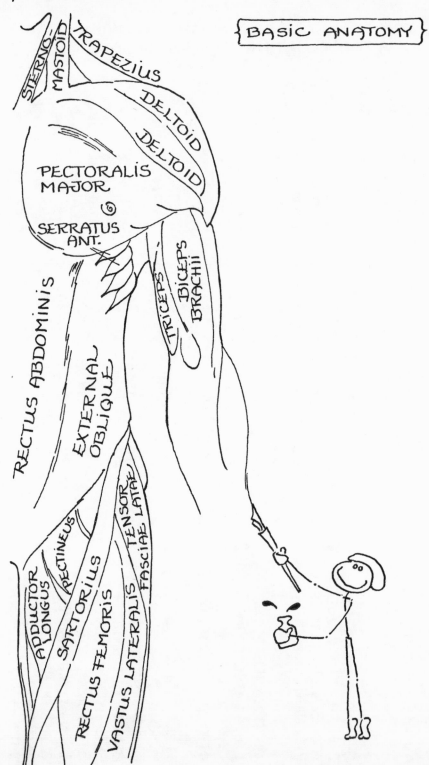

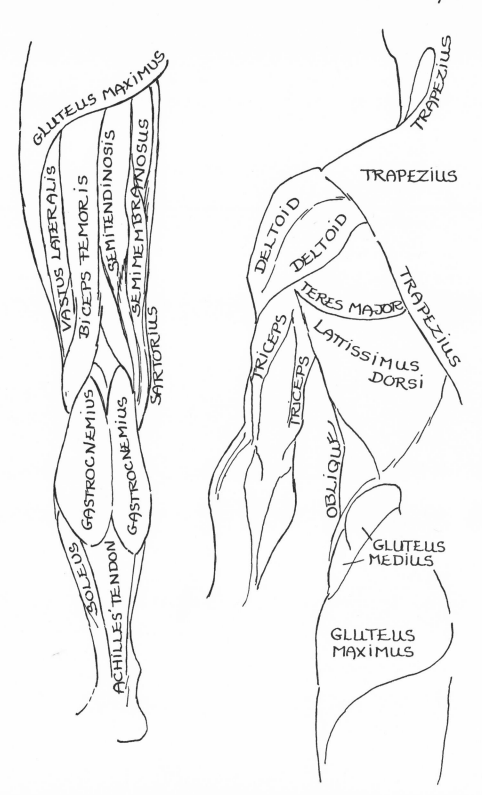

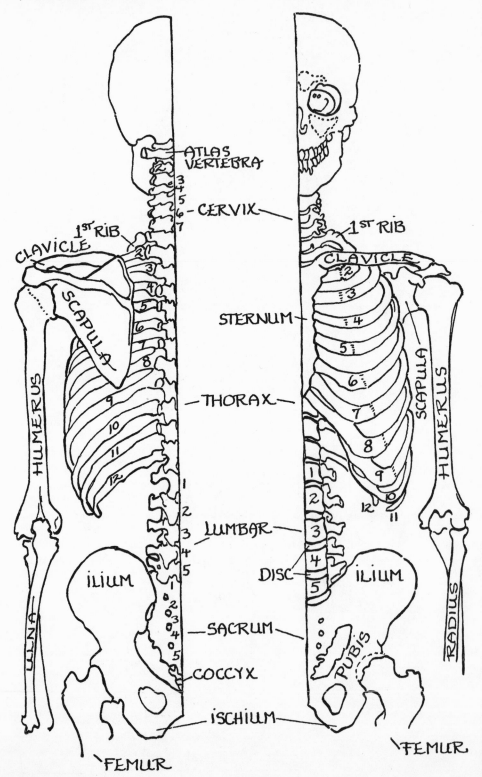

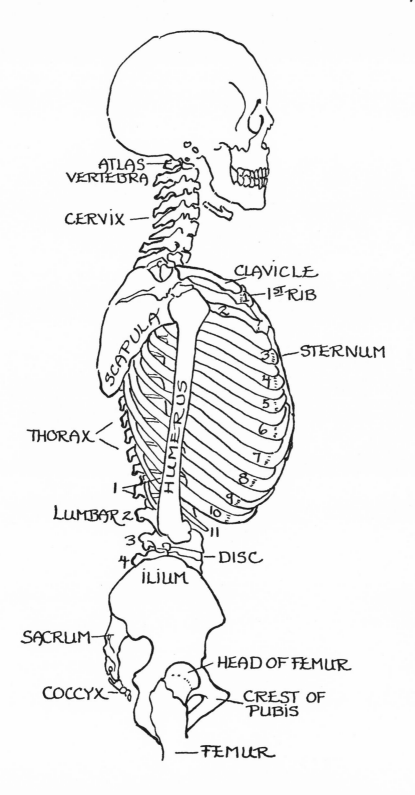

## { THE ART OF BREATHING }

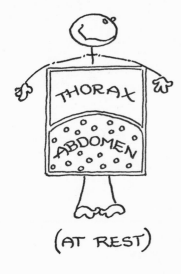

(AT REST)

THE MUSCULAR MEMBRANE OF THE DIAPHRAGM ARISES FROM THE STERNUM, THE LOWER RIBS AND THE LUMBAR VERTEBRAE... IT PARTIALLY SEPARATES THE THORACIC AND ABDOMINAL CAVITIES (CREATING A FLEXIBLE FLOOR FOR THE THORAX AND A FLEXIBLE CEILING FOR THE ABDOMEN)... AT REST, THE DIAPHRAGM IS A DOMED STRUCTURE ARCHED UP INTO THE CHEST...

FOR EFFICIENT INHALATION – RELAX THE ABDOMINAL WALL AND ALLOW THE VISCERA TO DISTEND SLIGHTLY, CREATING ADDITIONAL SPACE FOR THE DIAPHRAGM TO DROP AND FLATTEN... THE LOWER POSITION OF DIAPHRAGM CREATES A LARGER CHEST CAPACITY AND A REDUCTION OF AIR PRESSURE IN THE LUNGS...FRESH AIR IS BROUGHT INTO THE CHEST BY A VACUUM-TYPE PULL... THE DIAPHRAGM, DURING ITS DOWNSTROKE, WILL GENTLY MASSAGE THE ABDOMINAL VISCERA (IMPROVING DIGESTION AND CIRCULATION)... IF THE ABDOMINAL MUSCLES ARE HELD TIGHT DURING INHALATION, THE VISCERA ARE LOCKED IN PLACE AND THE DIAPHRAGM IS UNABLE TO DROP DOWN... BREATHING MUST THEN TAKE PLACE IN THE NARROWER, MORE RIGID AREAS OF THE UPPER CHEST.

(INHALATION)

{ THE ART OF BREATHING }

FOR EFFICIENT EXHALATION—
GENTLY TIGHTEN ABDOMINAL
WALL PULLING VISCERA
IN AND UP (THE
DIAPHRAGM WILL RECOIL
TO ITS DOMED POSITION)...
RELAX THE CHEST AND
DROP THE WEIGHT OF THE
RIBS ONTO THE LUNGS...

THE ENTIRE CYCLE SHOULD
BE SMOOTH, GENTLE, AND
RHYTHMIC.

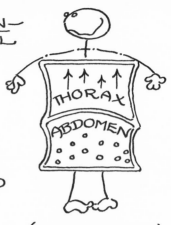

(EXHALATION)

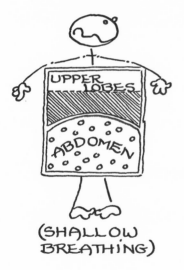

(SHALLOW
BREATHING)

THE HABIT OF SHALLOW AND
NARROW BREATHING :
ALLOWS THE DIAPHRAGM
AND THE RIB MUSCLES TO
GROW WEAK ; DEPRIVES
THE ABDOMINAL AND THE
THORACIC VISCERA OF
NECESSARY STIMULATION ;
ALLOWS INCOMING STALE
AIR, INFECTION AND
POLLUTION TO SETTLE
UNCHALLANGED IN THE
LOWER LUNGS ; LEAVES
THE BLOOD HUNGRY FOR
OXYGEN AND BURDENED
WITH USELESS RESIDUE...

TO UNDERSTAND AND USE THE BREATH
WISELY IS TO DRINK FROM THE ENDLESS
COSMIC SEA OF REFRESHING, SOOTHING,
HEALING ENERGY.

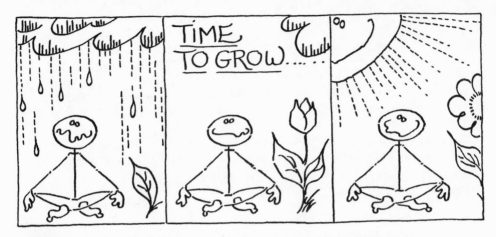

THE FOLLOWING 6-LEVEL PROGRAM IS OFFERED AS NOURISHMENT FOR YOUR CONTINUING GROWTH-MIND, BODY, SPIRIT....

BEFORE BEGINNING THE PROGRAM, <u>MEMORIZE</u> THE <u>BASIC TECHNIQUE</u> (PP 42-45) AND THE <u>BASIC POSITIONS</u> (PP 38-41).... CAREFULLY REVIEW THESE PAGES EACH TIME YOU ADVANCE TO A NEW LEVEL... SYMBOLS REPRESENTING THE BASIC TECHNIQUE ARE REPEATED THROUGHOUT THE BOOK TO KEEP THE TECHNIQUE FRESH IN YOUR MIND...

BEGIN AT LEVEL 1 AND PROGRESS THROUGH LEVEL 5.... ADVANCE TO THE NEXT LEVEL ONLY WHEN YOU ARE ABLE TO DO AND HOLD EACH POSE IN YOUR PRESENT LEVEL AS SUGGESTED... AT LEVEL 6 YOU WILL BE ABLE TO CREATE YOUR OWN LESSON PLANS ....

EACH OF THE 6 LEVELS IS DIVIDED INTO 2 SEPARATE SESSIONS:
1. DEEP BREATHING AND/OR A SALUTATION (THIS BRIEF SESSION IS IDEALLY, BUT NOT NECESSARILY, DONE BEFORE BREAKFAST)...
2. A COMPLETE PRACTICE SESSION (TO BE DONE AT A TIME THAT IS CONVENIENT AND COMFORTABLE FOR YOU)...

DO NOT REARRANGE THE CATEGORIES OF POSES, OR THE POSES WITHIN A CATEGORY....

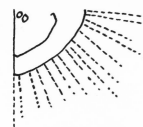

MOST OF THE PRACTICE SESSIONS INCLUDE THE FOLLOWING CATEGORIES:

1. <u>STRETCHING BREATHS</u> (TO PREPARE THE HEART AND LUNGS)...
2. <u>STANDING STRETCHES</u> (TO PREPARE THE MUSCLES AND TO FOCUS THE ATTENTION)...
3. <u>BALANCE</u> ON BOTH LEGS...
4. <u>BALANCE</u> ON 1 LEG...
5. A GENTLE <u>TRANSITION POSE</u> (TO PRERARE FOR FLOOR WORK)...
6. "<u>SMALL POSES</u>" THAT DO NOT INVOLVE THE TOTAL SPINE (EYES AND FACE, NECK, ARMS AND SHOULDERS, ANKLES AND FEET, LEGS)...
7. <u>FORWARD STRETCHES</u>...
8. <u>ABDOMINAL STRENGTHENING POSES</u>...
9. <u>LATERAL STRETCHES</u>...
10. <u>SPINAL TWISTS</u>...
11. <u>BACKWARD BENDING POSES</u>...
12. <u>INVERTED POSES</u>...
13. <u>QUIET BREATHING</u> AND <u>RELAXATION</u>...

TRY TO COMPLETE THE FULL PRACTICE SESSION AT LEAST 4 TIMES A WEEK...DO THE EARLY MORNING SESSION DAILY.... YOU MAY ABBREVIATE ANY OF THE FIRST 5 LEVELS BY DOING ONLY THOSE POSES MARKED WITH AN *....LEVEL 6 MAY BE SHORTENED BY OMITTING THE "SMALL POSES" CATEGORY....

IF YOU HAVE MISSED YOUR DAILY PRACTICE FOR MORE THAN A MONTH, BEGIN AGAIN AT LEVEL 1...

THE <u>VERY GENTLE LEVEL</u> IS PROVIDED FOR STUDENTS NOT ACCUSTOMED TO EXERCISE, OR STUDENTS RECOVERING FROM AN ILLNESS (GET YOUR DOCTOR'S OK)...

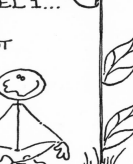

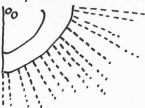

THE "MINI-POSES" (PP 63-67) ARE TO BE REMOVED FROM THE BOOK FOR USE AT YOUR DESK, IN A CAR, A MOTEL ROOM, A STUCK ELEVATOR ...

THE SUGGESTIONS ON PAGES 58-62 ARE OFFERED AS YOGIC TOOLS TO BE USED IN DEALING CREATIVELY WITH CERTAIN CHALLENGES (INSOMNIA, ANGER, PAIN) ...

EXPERIMENT WITH PASSIVE MEDITATION (P. 53), CREATIVE MEDITATION (P. 55), AND DEEP RELAXATION (P. 52) TO SELECT A DAILY PRACTICE TIME THAT SEEMS MOST EFFECTIVE...

STRETCH ONLY AS FAR INTO EACH POSE AS YOU WOULD INTO YOUR NATURAL MORNING STRETCH... HOLD A POSE ONLY AS LONG AS YOU ARE ABLE TO CONTROL THE TECHNIQUE, THE BREATHING, THE FOCUS ....

YOUR OWN COMMON SENSE AND INTUITIVE JUDGEMENT ARE IMPORTANT FACTORS IN THIS OR ANY OTHER PROGRAM YOU SELECT... AVOID SETTING GOALS AND DEADLINES FOR YOURSELF... UNFOLD NATURALLY AND ENJOY EACH STAGE OF YOUR GROWTH.. IMPATIENCE IS AS SENSELESS AS TEARING OPEN A ROSEBUD TO SEE HOW IT WILL LOOK IN FULL BLOOM. ...

THE LENGTH OF HOLDS AND THE NUMBER OF REPETITIONS ARE SUGGESTED AS THE MAXIMUM TIME TO BE SPENT IN THE HOLD - AND THE MAXIMUM NUMBER OF REPETITIONS.

THE POSES THAT MAKE UP A SALUTATION SHOULD FLOW TOGETHER SMOOTHLY.. HOLD EACH POSE JUST LONG ENOUGH TO FOCUS.

# VERY GENTLE

| NAME OF POSTURE | PAGE | HOLD $\overset{\circ}{R}$ REPEAT |
|---|---|---|
| WINGED BREATH.... | 105 | ....5 TIMES |
| TEMPLE BREATH.... | 72 | ... 5 TIMES |
| *STRETCH BREATH, FORWARD......... | 71 | .....5 TIMES |
| *HAND-TO-FOOT 1....... | 73 | ....15 SECONDS |
| SHOULDER SHIFT...... | 74 | ...15 SEC., EACH SIDE |
| *TRIANGLE 1.......... | 75 | ....15 SEC., EACH SIDE |
| *WISE MAN POSE...... | 76 | ....15 SEC., EACH SIDE |
| SMALL MOUNTAIN..... | 77 | ....15 SECONDS |
| TREE 1 .............. | 79 | .....15 SEC., EACH SIDE |
| *WIND 1 .............. | 80 | .....15 SEC., EACH SIDE |
| CLOCK ................ | 75 | .....1 TIME, EACH WAY |
| CLENCH............... | 81 | .....3 TIMES |
| *HEAD TILT 1 AND 2.. | 82, 72 | ...3 TIMES, EACH |
| SHOULDER LIFT....... | 83 | ....5 TIMES |
| DRAGONFLY .......... | 84 | .....3 TIMES, EACH ARM |
| WRIST BEND.......... | 86 | .....3 TIMES |
| *KNEE STRETCH...... | 88 | .....15 SEC., EACH KNEE |
| *HEEL-TO-CHEST...... | 89 | .....15 SEC., EACH SIDE |
| *HEAD-TO-KNEE 1..... | 90 | ....15 SEC., EACH SIDE |
| HALF TORTOISE ..... | 91 | .....15 SECONDS |
| PELVIC TILT......... | 92 | ...15 SECONDS |
| *ATLAS BEND........ | 93 | ....15 SEC., EACH SIDE |
| *TWIST 1.............. | 94 | ....15 SEC., EACH SIDE |
| *COBRA 1............. | 95 | ....15 SECONDS |
| *HALF LOCUST 1...... | 96 | ....15 SEC., EACH SIDE |
| CAMEL 1............ | 90 | ....15 SECONDS |
| *BRIDGE 1 OR 2....... | 88, 97 | ...15 SECONDS |
| *WALL REST........... | 98 | ....60 SECONDS |
| OR FOLDED LEAF........ | 98 | ....30 SECONDS |

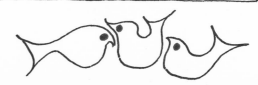

# LEVEL # 1

| NAME OF POSTURE | PAGE | HOLD $\overset{O}{R}$ REPEAT |
|---|---|---|

| | | |
|---|---|---|
| WINGED BREATH .... | 105 | ...5 TIMES |
| STRETCH BREATH,<br>  FORWARD ........... | 71 | ...5 TIMES |

| | | |
|---|---|---|
| *STRETCH BREATH,<br>  FORWARD ........... | 71 | ....5 TIMES |
| TEMPLE BREATH.... | 72 | ....5 TIMES |
| *HAND-TO-FOOT 1..... | 73 | ....30 SECONDS |
| *TRIANGLE 1 ........ | 75 | ....30 SEC., EACH SIDE |
| *WISE MAN POSE..... | 76 | ....30 SEC., EACH SIDE |
| SMALL MOUNTAIN.... | 77 | ....30 SECONDS |
| *UNEVEN ............. | 78 | ....30 SECONDS |
| *WIND 1............... | 80 | ....30 SEC., EACH LEG |
| CLOCK............... | 75 | ....1 TIME, EACH WAY |
| CLENCH............. | 81 | ....3 TIMES |
| *HEAD TILT 1 AND 2.. | 82, 72.. | 3 TIMES, EACH |
| ARM TURN........... | 85 | .... 3 TIMES |
| ELBOW LOCK........ | 78 | ....30 SECONDS |
| *KNEE STRETCH.... | 88 | ....30 SEC., EACH KNEE |
| CRADLE............. | 99 | ....30 SEC., EACH LEG |
| *HEAD-TO-KNEE 1.. | 90 | ....30 SEC., EACH SIDE |
| *BACK STRETCH 1... | 100 | ....30 SECONDS |
| HALF TORTOISE..... | 91 | ....30 SECONDS |
| *SPINAL COLUMN 1... | 101 | ....30 SECONDS |
| *ATLAS BEND........ | 93 | ....30 SEC., EACH SIDE |
| *SPINAL TWIST 2 ..... | 85 | ....30 SEC., EACH SIDE |
| *COBRA 2........... | 102 | ....30 SECONDS |
| *HALF LOCUST 1 ..... | 96 | ....30 SEC., EACH LEG |
| PELVIC STRETCH... | 103 | ...30 SECONDS |
| *STANDING REST..... | 104 | ....60 SECONDS |
| ABDOMINAL BREATH. | 47 | ...5 BREATHS |
| MASTER BREATH.... | 49 | ....UP TO 5 MINUTES |

# LEVEL # II

| NAME OF POSTURE | PAGE | HOLD & REPEAT |
|---|---|---|

| | | |
|---|---|---|
| WINGED BREATH....105...5 TIMES | | |
| STRETCH BREATH, | | |
| FORWARD..........71....5 TIMES | | |

| | | |
|---|---|---|
| *STRETCH BREATH, | | |
| FORWARD.........71....5 TIMES | | |
| STRETCH BREATH, | | |
| LATERAL..........87.....5 TIMES | | |
| *HAND-TO-FOOT 1....73.....30 SECONDS | | |
| *INTENSE SIDE ST....106....30 SEC., EACH SIDE | | |
| *TRIANGLE 1........75....30 SEC., EACH SIDE | | |
| *MOON POSE.........107....30 SEC., EACH SIDE | | |
| *THIGH POSE.........77.....30 SECONDS | | |
| EAGLE 1............108....30 SEC., EACH SIDE | | |
| TREE 2..........113....30 SEC., EACH SIDE | | |
| *WIND 2.............80.....60 SECONDS | | |
| SUN, RISING.......109....30 SEC., EACH SIDE | | |
| *YOGA SEAL..........79....30 SECONDS | | |
| ANKLE BALANCE 1.111....30 SEC., EACH FOOT | | |
| *KNEE STRETCH.....88.....30 SEC., EACH KNEE | | |
| LOTUS BLOSSOMING...93....30 SEC., EACH LEG | | |
| *HEAD-TO-KNEE 2....112....30 SEC., EACH SIDE | | |
| STAR 1..............113....30 SECONDS | | |
| *BACK STRETCH 2..114....30 SECONDS | | |
| *ATLAS BEND........93.....30 SEC., EACH SIDE | | |
| *SPINAL COLUMN 2..99.....30 SECONDS | | |
| *SPINAL TWIST 3...114.....30 SEC., EACH SIDE | | |
| *COBRA 2...........102...30 SECONDS | | |
| *HALF LOCUST 2.......96....20 SECONDS | | |
| BACKWARD BEND..115....30 SECONDS | | |
| *TRANQUILITY........116....60 SECONDS | | |
| *MID-CHEST BREATH..47....5 BREATHS | | |
| SURFACE BREATH...47...UP TO 5 MINUTES | | |

# LEVEL · III

| NAME OF POSTURE | PAGE | HOLD OR REPEAT |
|---|---|---|

| WINGED BREATH..... 105 .....5 TIMES | | |
|---|---|---|

SALUTATION TO THE SUN (STEPS 1, 3, 4, 5, 6, 9, 12, 15, 16, 17, AND 19)..UP TO 3 TIMES
150

| NAME OF POSTURE | PAGE | HOLD OR REPEAT |
|---|---|---|
| *STRETCH BREATH, FORWARD..........71 .....10 TIMES | | |
| *HAND-TO-FOOT 1.....73 .....30 SECONDS | | |
| *INTENSE SIDE ST.... 106.....30 SEC., EACH SIDE | | |
| OPEN BOOK .......118 .....30 SECONDS | | |
| *HALF MOON 1......119 .....30 SEC., EACH SIDE | | |
| *TOE POSE 1........120.....30 SECONDS | | |
| EAGLE 2 .............82 ....30 SEC., EACH SIDE | | |
| LORD OF DANCERS...121 ....30 SEC., EACH SIDE | | |
| *WIND POSE 2 .......80.....60 SECONDS | | |
| LION .................122....3 TIMES | | |
| *NECK ROLL.......122....3 TIMES, EACH WAY | | |
| *COWHEAD 1.........123 ....30 SEC., EACH SIDE | | |
| ARM MOTION .......110 ....30 SECONDS | | |
| ANKLE BALANCE 2.. 111 ....30 SECONDS | | |
| HALF LOTUS........124 ....30 SEC., EACH SIDE | | |
| *COBBLER .........125....30 SECONDS | | |
| RIGHT ANGLE POSE..127....30 SEC., EACH LEG | | |
| *HEAD-TO-KNEE 3.... 74....30 SEC., EACH SIDE | | |
| *BACK STRETCH 2..114...30 SECONDS | | |
| SEPARATE LEG ST. ...109.....30 SECONDS | | |
| *UPWARD LEG ST. ...126 ....20 SEC., EACH ANGLE | | |
| *HEAD-TO-KNEE 5.....128....30 SEC., EACH SIDE | | |
| *SPINAL TWIST 4..... 81 ....30 SEC., EACH SIDE | | |
| *DOG TO MOON.......129....30 SECONDS | | |
| *HALF LOCUST 2 ......96....20 SECONDS | | |
| *BOW 1 ...............101....30 SECONDS | | |
| *PLOUGH............131....60 SECONDS | | |
| *COMPLETE BREATH... 48....5 TIMES | | |
| PERFECT BREATH.... 50....UP TO 5 MINUTES | | |

# LEVEL · IV

| NAME OF POSTURE | PAGE | HOLD & REPEAT |
|---|---|---|

TEMPLE BREATH..... 72 ... 5 TIMES
WINGED BREATH ..... 105 ... 5 TIMES
SALUTATION TO THE SUN (STEPS 1, 2, 3, 4, 5,
6, 9, 10, 11, 12, 15, 16, 17, 18, 19)....UP TO 3
TIMES                150

*STRETCH BREATH,
　　FORWARD......... 71 .... 10 TIMES
*HAND-TO-FOOT 2 ..... 117 ... 30 SECONDS
　OPEN BOOK ......... 118 ... 30 SECONDS
*TRIANGLE 2......... 132 ... 30 SECONDS
*TOE POSE 1 OR 2.... 120 ... 30 SECONDS

　HALF SQUAT, 1 LEG.. 133 ... 30 SEC., EACH SIDE
　HEAD-TO-KNEE 6.... 134 ... 30 SEC., EACH SIDE

*WIND 2............... 80 ... 60 SECONDS

　LION ............... 122 ... 3 TIMES
*NECK STRETCH..... 133 ... 30 SECONDS
*COWHEAD 2......... 123 ... 30 SEC., EACH SIDE
　INCLINED PLANE.... 104 ... 30 SECONDS
　ANKLE BALANCE 2... 111 ... 30 SECONDS
*GENTLE POSE ...... 124 ... 30 SECONDS
　HERON ............. 135 ... 30 SEC., EACH SIDE
　SEATED FROG........ 94 ... 30 SECONDS

*HEAD-TO-KNEE 4.... 92 ... 30 SEC., EACH SIDE
*STAR 2............... 86 ... 30 SECONDS
　3 LIMBS ............ 136 ... 30 SEC., EACH SIDE

*BOAT WITH OARS..... 95 ... 30 SECONDS

*HEAD-TO-KNEE 5.... 128 ... 30 SEC., EACH SIDE

*SPINAL TWIST 5...... 137 ... 30 SEC., EACH SIDE

*SERPENT........... 108 ... 30 SECONDS
*BOW 2............... 138 ... 30 SEC., EACH SIDE
　CAMEL 2............ 139 ... 30 SECONDS
　FISH............... 129 ... 30 SECONDS

*KNEE-TO-EAR....... 140 ... 60 SECONDS

*SUN BREATH........ 46 ... 5 BREATHS
*MOON BREATH....... 50 ... 5 BREATHS

# LEVEL ◦ V

| NAME OF POSTURE | PAGE | HOLD $\frac{O}{R}$ REPEAT |
|---|---|---|

TEMPLE BREATH..... 72.... 5 TIMES
WINGED BREATH .....105 ...5 TIMES
SALUTATION TO THE SUN (COMPLETE)...
     UP TO 3 TIMES 150

*STRETCH BREATH,
     FORWARD AND.... 71 ....5 TIMES
* LATERAL........... 87 ....5 TIMES

*HAND-TO-FOOT 2 .....117..... 30 SECONDS
*HALF MOON 2 .......110 ...20 SECONDS
 POWERFUL POSE ....141 ...30 SEC., EACH SIDE
*LATERAL ANGLE ST...142 ...30 SEC., EACH SIDE

 EAGLE 2..............82....30 SEC., EACH SIDE
 BOW, STANDING......125....30 SEC., EACH SIDE

*WIND 2 ..............80 ...60 SECONDS

 LION.................122... 3 TIMES
*NECK ROLL .........122... 3 TIMES, EACH WAY
*PENDANT..............115....30 SECONDS
*FULL LOTUS.........143...30 SEC., EACH SIDE
 PILLAR...............89...30 SEC., EACH LEG
 BALANCED BACK ST...103...30 SECONDS

*HEAD-TO-KNEE 4......92...30 SEC., EACH SIDE
*BACK STRETCH 2 ....114...30 SECONDS
 TORTOISE ...........84...30 SECONDS
 RABBIT..............97...30 SECONDS

* SMALL BOAT.........126...30 SECONDS

* GATE LATCH........144...30 SEC., EACH SIDE

* SPINAL TWIST 6.......83 ..30 SEC., EACH SIDE

*SERPENT..............108...30 SECONDS
*HALF LOCUST 2 .......96...20 SECONDS
*BOW 1................101...30 SECONDS
 SLEEPING WARRIOR.145...30 SECONDS

*SHOULDER STAND.....146..60 SECONDS

*ALTERNATE NOSTRIL..49...5 CYCLES
 CALM BREATH........49...UP TO 5 MINUTES

# LEVEL # VI

| NAME OF POSTURE | PAGE | HOLD $\overset{O}{R}$ REPEAT |
|---|---|---|

### DEEP BREATHING + A SALUTATION
(SELECT 1 FROM EACH GROUP)

| | | |
|---|---|---|
| TEMPLE BREATH...72 | | 5 TIMES |
| WINGED BREATH...105 | | 5 TIMES |
| STRETCH BREATH, FORWARD...71 | | 5 TIMES |
| SUN SALUTATION....150 | | UP TO 12 TIMES |
| MOON SALUTATION...153 | | UP TO 12 TIMES |

1.

### STRETCHING - CLEANSING BREATHING
(SELECT 1 FROM EACH GROUP)

| | | |
|---|---|---|
| WINGED BREATH....105 | | 5 TIMES |
| TEMPLE BREATH.....72 | | 5 TIMES |
| STRETCH BREATH, LATERAL...87 | | 5 TIMES |
| STRETCH BREATH, FORWARD...71 | | 5 TIMES |

2.

### STANDING STRETCHES
(SELECT 1 FROM EACH GROUP)

| | | |
|---|---|---|
| HAND-TO-FOOT 1...73 | | 30 SECONDS |
| HAND-TO-FOOT 2...117 | | 30 SECONDS |
| OPEN BOOK........118 | | 30 SECONDS |
| TRIANGLE 1........75 | | 30 SEC., EACH SIDE |
| TRIANGLE 2.......132 | | 30 SEC., EACH SIDE |
| HALF MOON 1......119 | | 30 SEC., EACH SIDE |
| WISE MAN POSE....76 | | 30 SEC., EACH SIDE |
| MOON POSE.......107 | | 30 SEC., EACH SIDE |
| HALF MOON 2.....110 | | 20 SECONDS |
| INTENSE SIDE ST..106 | | 30 SEC., EACH SIDE |
| POWERFUL POSE..141 | | 30 SEC., EACH SIDE |
| LATERAL ANGLE..142 | | 30 SEC., EACH SIDE |

# LEVEL·VI

| NAME OF POSTURE | PAGE | HOLD ᴼ/ᴿ REPEAT |
|---|---|---|

**3.**

| BALANCE-ON BOTH LEGS (SELECT 1 FROM EACH GROUP) | | |
|---|---|---|
| UNEVEN | 78 | 30 SECONDS |
| THIGH POSE | 77 | 30 SECONDS |
| TOE POSE 1 | 120 | 30 SECONDS |
| TOE POSE 2 | 120 | 30 SECONDS |

**4.**

| BALANCE-ON 1 LEG (SELECT 1 FROM EACH GROUP) | | |
|---|---|---|
| TREE 2 | 113 | 30 SEC., EACH SIDE |
| LORD ᴼ/ᶠ DANCERS | 121 | 30 SEC., EACH SIDE |
| EAGLE 2 | 82 | 30 SEC., EACH SIDE |
| HALF SQUAT, 1 LEG | 133 | 30 SEC., EACH SIDE |
| POSE ᴼ/ᶠ KNOWLEDGE | 149 | 30 SEC., EACH SIDE |
| HEAD-TO-KNEE 6 | 134 | 30 SEC., EACH SIDE |
| FULL MOON | 148 | 30 SEC., EACH SIDE |
| BOW, STANDING | 125 | 30 SEC., EACH SIDE |

**5.**

| TRANSITION POSE (SELECT 1) | | |
|---|---|---|
| WIND 1 | 80 | 30 SEC., EACH SIDE |
| WIND 2 | 80 | 60 SECONDS |
| FOLDED LEAF | 98 | 60 SECONDS |

**6.**

| SMALL POSES (SELECT 1 FROM EACH GROUP) | | |
|---|---|---|
| CLOCK | 75 | 2 TIMES, EACH WAY |
| CLENCH | 81 | 3 TIMES |
| LION | 122 | 3 TIMES |
| NECK ROLL | 122 | 3 TIMES, EACH WAY |
| NECK STRETCH | 133 | 30 SECONDS |
| COWHEAD 1 | 123 | 30 SEC., EACH SIDE |
| COWHEAD 2 | 123 | 30 SEC., EACH SIDE |
| YOGA SEAL | 79 | 30 SECONDS |
| INCLINED PLANE | 104 | 30 SECONDS |
| PENDANT | 115 | 30 SECONDS |

# LEVEL VI

| NAME OF POSTURE | PAGE | HOLD $\overset{o}{R}$ REPEAT |
|---|---|---|

**6.**

## SMALL POSES (CONTINUED)

| | | |
|---|---|---|
| KNEE STRETCH | 88 | 30 SEC., EACH SIDE |
| HALF LOTUS | 124 | 30 SEC., EACH SIDE |
| FULL LOTUS | 143 | 30 SEC., EACH SIDE |
| CRADLE | 99 | 30 SEC., EACH SIDE |
| COBBLER | 125 | 30 SECONDS |
| GENTLE | 124 | 30 SECONDS |
| LOTUS BLOSSOMING | 93 | 30 SEC., EACH LEG |
| RIGHT ANGLE | 127 | 30 SEC., EACH LEG |
| HERON | 135 | 30 SEC., EACH SIDE |
| PILLAR | 89 | 30 SEC., EACH SIDE |
| BALANCED BACK ST. | 163 | 30 SECONDS |
| RAISED THUNDEBOLT | 135 | 30 SECONDS |

**7.**

## FORWARD STRETCHES
## (SELECT 1 FROM EACH GROUP)

| | | |
|---|---|---|
| HEAD-TO-KNEE 1 | 90 | 30 SEC., EACH SIDE |
| HEAD-TO-KNEE 2 | 112 | 30 SEC., EACH SIDE |
| HEAD-TO-KNEE 3 | 74 | 30 SEC., EACH SIDE |
| HEAD-TO-KNEE 4 | 92 | 30 SEC., EACH SIDE |
| 3 LIMBS | 136 | 30 SEC., EACH SIDE |
| BACK STRETCH 2 | 114 | 60 SECONDS |
| STAR 2 | 86 | 30 SECONDS |
| TORTOISE | 84 | 30 SECONDS |
| HALF TORTOISE | 91 | 30 SECONDS |
| RABBIT | 97 | 30 SECONDS |

**8.**

## ABDOMINAL STRENGTHENING POSE (DO 1)

| | | |
|---|---|---|
| SPINAL COLUMN 2 | 99 | 30 SECONDS |
| UPWARD LEG ST. | 126 | 20 SEC., EACH ANGLE |
| SMALL BOAT | 126 | 30 SECONDS |
| BOAT WITH OARS | 95 | 30 SECONDS |

# LEVEL · VI

| NAME OF POSTURE | PAGE | HOLD OR REPEAT |
|---|---|---|

**9.**

| LATERAL STRETCH (SELECT 1) | | |
|---|---|---|
| HEAD-TO-KNEE 5 | 128 | 30 SEC., EACH SIDE |
| ATLAS BEND | 93 | 30 SEC., EACH SIDE |
| GATE LATCH | 144 | 30 SEC., EACH SIDE |

**10.**

| FULL SPINAL TWIST (SELECT 1) | | |
|---|---|---|
| SPINAL TWIST 2 | 85 | 30 SEC., EACH SIDE |
| SPINAL TWIST 3 | 114 | 30 SEC., EACH SIDE |
| SPINAL TWIST 4 | 81 | 30 SEC., EACH SIDE |
| SPINAL TWIST 5 | 137 | 30 SEC., EACH SIDE |
| SPINAL TWIST 6 | 83 | 30 SEC., EACH SIDE |

**11.**

| BACKWARD BENDS (SELECT 1 FROM EACH GROUP) | | |
|---|---|---|
| COBRA 2 | 102 | 30 SECONDS |
| SERPENT | 108 | 30 SECONDS |
| DOG, FACE TO MOON | 129 | 30 SECONDS |
| MONKEY | 130 | 30 SEC., EACH SIDE |
| HALF LOCUST 1 | 96 | 30 SEC., EACH LEG |
| HALF LOCUST 2 | 96 | 20 SECONDS |
| BOW 1 | 101 | 30 SECONDS |
| BOW 2 | 138 | 30 SEC., EACH SIDE |
| FULL LOCUST | 134 | 30 SECONDS |
| PELVIC STRETCH | 103 | 30 SECONDS |
| CAMEL 2 | 139 | 30 SECONDS |
| SLEEPING WARRIOR | 145 | 30 SECONDS |
| FISH | 129 | 30 SECONDS |
| SLEEPING FROG | 147 | 30 SECONDS |

**12.**

| INVERTED POSE (SELECT 1) | | |
|---|---|---|
| TRANQUILITY | 116 | 60 SECONDS |
| PLOUGH | 131 | 60 SECONDS |
| KNEE-TO-EAR | 140 | 60 SECONDS |
| SHOULDER STAND | 146 | 60 SECONDS |
| WALL REST | 98 | 60 SECONDS |

# LEVEL · VI

| NAME OF POSTURE | PAGE | HOLD $\frac{O}{R}$ REPEAT |
|---|---|---|

13.

| QUIET BREATHING + RELAXATION (SELECT 1 FROM EACH GROUP) | | |
|---|---|---|
| SIPPING BREATH... | 51 | ...5 TIMES |
| SUN BREATH....... | 46 | ...5 TIMES |
| MOON BREATH..... | 50 | ...5 TIMES |
| ALTERNATE NOSTRIL. | 49 | ...5 TIMES |
| RHYTHMIC.......... | 50 | ...5 TIMES |
| MASTER BREATH.... | 49 | ...UP TO 5 MINUTES |
| SURFACE BREATH.... | 47 | ...UP TO 5 MINUTES |
| PERFECT BREATH... | 50 | ...UP TO 5 MINUTES |
| FLOWING BREATH... | 51 | ....UP TO 5 MINUTES |
| OR DEEP RELAXATION... | 52 | ...UP TO 5 MINUTES |

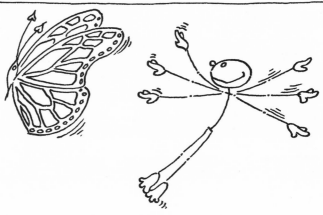

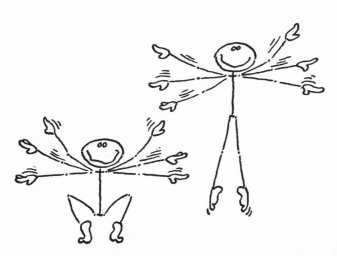

## {BASIC POSITIONS}

MOST OF THE ASANAS DESCRIBED IN THIS BOOK WILL BEGIN AND END IN ONE OF THE FOLLOWING BASIC POSITIONS:

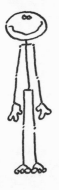

### STANDING POSE

1. GENTLY STRETCH TOP OF HEAD TOWARD CEILING...
2. RELAX SHOULDERS, ARMS...
3. KEEP LEGS STRAIGHT, BUT KNEES UNLOCKED...
4. DISTRIBUTE WEIGHT EVENLY BETWEEN BALL OF FOOT AND HEEL, BETWEEN BIG TOE AND LITTLE TOE...
5. PUSH STERNUM FORWARD ABOUT 1/2 INCH.

### SEATED POSE

1. SIT WITH BACK ERECT...
2. GENTLY STRETCH TOP OF HEAD TOWARD CEILING...
3. EXTEND LEGS FORWARD WITH INNER LEGS TOGETHER...
4. RELAX ARMS, SHOULDERS...
5. REST HANDS ON THIGHS.

### PRONE POSE

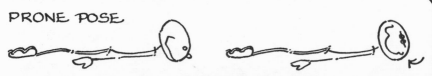

1. LIE FACE DOWN WITH ARMS STRAIGHT AND CLOSE TO BODY...
2. KEEP LEGS TOGETHER, TOES POINTED...
3. GENTLY PUSH TOP OF HEAD FORWARD (AWAY FROM HIPS)...
4. WHEN RESTING IN PRONE POSE, TURN HEAD AND REST ON CHEEK.

## {BASIC POSITIONS}

### EASY POSE

1. SIT STRAIGHT AND "TALL"...
2. CROSS ANKLES IN FRONT OF (AND CLOSE TO) BODY... DROP KNEES TO FLOOR...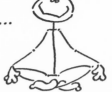
3. REST HANDS ON KNEES OR THIGHS...
4. RELAX ARMS, SHOULDERS...
5. PUSH STERNUM FORWARD ABOUT ½ INCH.

### SIDE-LYING POSE

1. LIE ON OUTER HIP AND OUTSIDE OF LOWER LEG...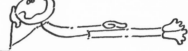
2. KEEP LEGS STRAIGHT AND INNER EDGES OF FEET TOGETHER...
3. REST SIDE OF HEAD IN HAND, ELBOW ON FLOOR...
4. PLACE OTHER PALM ON OUTSIDE OF UPPER THIGH.

### SPREAD FOOT POSE

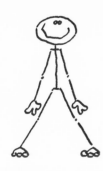

1. STAND TALL...
2. RELAX SHOULDERS, ARMS...
3. TAKE A WIDE SIDE-STEP (USUALLY 3 OR 4 FEET)...
4. KEEP INNER EDGES OF FEET PARALLEL...
5. LOCK KNEES, TIGHTEN THIGH MUSCLES.

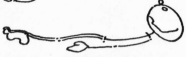

## BASIC POSITIONS

### SUPINE POSE

1. LIE ON BACK, FACE UP...
2. KEEP LEGS TOGETHER AND STRAIGHT...
3. TUCK STRAIGHT ARMS AGAINST SIDES...
4. REACH GENTLY TOWARD FEET TO PULL SHOULDERS AWAY FROM NECK.

### KNEELING POSE

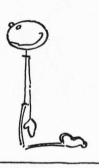

1. STAND ON KNEES...
2. PLACE KNEES AND FEET HIP-WIDTH APART...
3. RELAX ARMS BY SIDES...
4. KEEP SPINE ERECT.

### THUNDERBOLT POSE

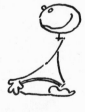

1. KNEEL, SITTING BACK ON HEELS...
2. KEEP KNEES, INNER THIGHS, TIPS OF BIG TOES TOGETHER...
3. RELAX ANKLES AND FEET, ALLOWING HEELS TO TURN OUT...
4. REST HANDS ON KNEES OR THIGHS...
5. SIT STRAIGHT AND TALL.

{BASIC POSITIONS}

## HEROIC POSE

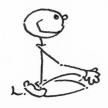

1. SIT STRAIGHT AND "TALL"...
2. CROSS THIGHS IN FRONT OF BODY, PLACING 1 KNEE DIRECTLY OVER OTHER...
3. BRING RIGHT HEEL TO OUTER LEFT HIP AND LEFT HEEL TO OUTER RIGHT HIP (DO NOT SIT ON HEELS)...
4. REST HANDS ON UPPER KNEE.

## ANGLED FOOT POSE

1. STAND "TALL"...
2. RELAX SHOULDERS, ARMS...
3. TAKE A WIDE SIDE-STEP... (3 OR 4 FEET WITH INNER EDGES OF FEET PARALLEL)...
4. TURN TOES EITHER RIGHT OR LEFT (PIVOT ON HEELS)...
5. PLACE INNER EDGE OF FORWARD FOOT PARALLEL TO FRONT WALL...TURN BACK FOOT AT LEAST HALFWAY AROUND SO STRETCH IS FELT DOWN ACHILLES' TENDON INTO HEEL...
6. KEEP HEELS IN LINE WITH EACH OTHER.

## SPONGE POSE

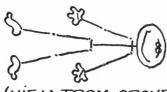

(VIEW FROM ABOVE)

1. LIE ON BACK...
2. REST ARMS ON FLOOR ABOUT 12 INCHES FROM BODY (PALMS UP)...
3. SEPARATE FEET HIP-WIDTH APART (ALLOW TOES TO TURN OUT)...
4. RELAX ENTIRE BODY.

## {BASIC TECHNIQUE}

YOGA IS MEANT TO COMPLEMENT, NOT TO REPLACE, REGULAR MEDICAL CHECK-UPS... ASK FOR YOUR DOCTOR'S APPROVAL AND SUGGESTIONS BEFORE BEGINNING ANY YOGA OR PHYSICAL FITNESS PROGRAM... THE DOCTOR SHOULD HELP PLAN A SPECIAL PROGRAM FOR YOU IF YOU ARE BEING TREATED FOR HEART OR LUNG DISEASE.

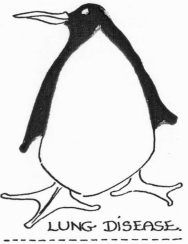

------------------------------------

THE REST AFTER A POSE SHOULD BE CONSIDERED AN IMPORTANT PART OF THAT POSE... CONTINUE TO FOCUS AND TO CONCENTRATE... DEEPLY RELAX EVERY MUSCLE NOT NECESSARY TO MAINTAIN REST POSITION... TAKE AT LEAST ③ COMPLETE BREATHS (P. 48).

------------------------------------

MOVE GRACEFULLY, SMOOTHLY, QUIETLY FROM THE FIRST TO THE LAST MOMENT OF EACH PRACTICE SESSION (THE SESSION THEN BECOMES 1 FLUID MOVEMENT INSTEAD OF A SERIES OF SEPARATE, UNCONNECTED POSES)... THE CONCENTRATION AND SERENITY OF 1 POSE SHOULD CREATE A FOUNDATION FOR THE FOLLOWING POSE.

## {BASIC TECHNIQUE}

BOTH THE BODY AND THE MIND MAY AT FIRST STUBBORNLY RESIST CHANGE...BE PATIENT... THE BODY-MIND-SPIRIT MUST UNFOLD NATURALLY, GRADUALLY, SLOWLY... NEVER FORCE THE BODY IN ANY WAY.

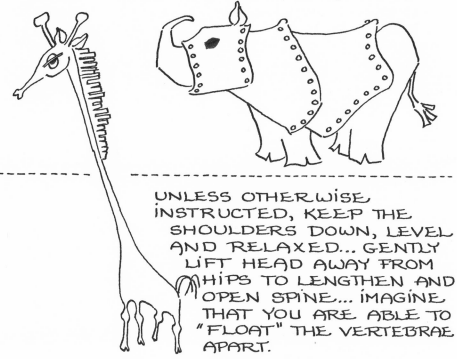

UNLESS OTHERWISE INSTRUCTED, KEEP THE SHOULDERS DOWN, LEVEL AND RELAXED... GENTLY LIFT HEAD AWAY FROM HIPS TO LENGTHEN AND OPEN SPINE... IMAGINE THAT YOU ARE ABLE TO "FLOAT" THE VERTEBRAE APART.

MOVE VERY SLOWLY DURING POSTURES...TAKE AT LEAST 5 SECONDS FOR EACH MAJOR CHANGE OF DIRECTION (KNEE TO CHEST, HEAD TO KNEE, HANDS BEHIND HEAD).

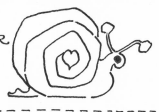

DO POSES ON AN EVEN, PADDED, NON-SKID SURFACE... USE A FOLDED TOWEL UNDER KNEES, ANKLES, OR SENSITIVE VERTEBRAE IF YOU NEED EXTRA PROTECTION...

{ BASIC TECHNIQUE }

PRACTICE THE ASANAS WITH EYES <u>OPEN</u>...
<u>FOCUS</u> (WITHOUT STRAIN) ON 1 SMALL
FIXED POINT DURING POSES AND RESTS...
A SUGGESTED LOCATION OF FOCUS IS
GIVEN WITH EACH INDIVIDUAL POSE...
CLOSE EYES WHEN FACE RESTS DIRECTLY
ON FLOOR OR
LEGS...EYES MAY
BE OPEN OR
CLOSED DURING
MEDITATION AND
DURING QUIET
BREATHING
EXERCISES.

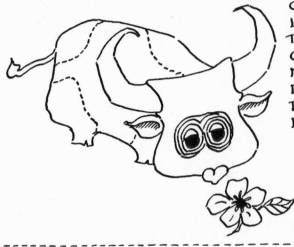

---

DURING EACH POSE <u>BREATHE</u> QUIETLY
AND <u>NATURALLY</u> THROUGH THE <u>NOSE</u>...DO
NOT HOLD YOUR BREATH OR FORCE AIR
INTO AREAS OF THE LUNGS INTENTIONALLY
SQUEEZED AND COMPRESSED BY POSE...
THE BREATH IS ALWAYS THE FOUNDATION OF
EACH POSE AND MUST, THEREFORE, BE
CONSTANTLY CHECKED AND REFINED...
SELECT LENGTH OF BREATH THAT IS MOST
COMFORTABLE... DURING FORWARD BENDING
AND STRETCHING KEEP EXHALATION LONGER
THAN INHALATION...SHALLOW-BREATHE
DURING BACK BENDING
POSES WHEN THE
BODY BALANCES ON
THE ABDOMEN (HALF
LOCUST, BOW).

## {BASIC TECHNIQUE}

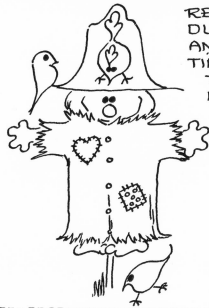

REMAIN ABSOLUTELY STILL DURING EACH HOLD ... ANY MOVEMENT AT THIS TIME SUBTRACTS FROM THE PHYSICAL AND MENTAL BENEFITS OF THE POSE... HOWEVER, SUBTLE, QUIET WORK CONTINUES DURING THE HOLD ... THE "INNER EYES" OF THE MIND CONSTANTLY EXPLORE AND REFINE THE INNER ENVIRONMENT.

--------------------------------

IT IS WISE DURING ANY STAGE OF PREGNANCY TO TAKE THIS BOOK WITH YOU TO THE DOCTOR TO HAVE YOUR CURRENT LESSON PLAN APPROVED... AVOID THE HALF LOCUST AND THE BOW DURING ALL 9 MONTHS (AND ANY OTHER POSE THAT PUTS PRESSURE ON THE UPPER UTERUS OR INTERFERES WITH BREATHING).

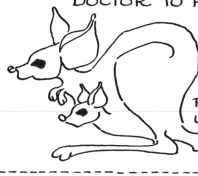

--------------------------------

DO NOT EAT FOR AT LEAST 2 HOURS BEFORE DOING YOGA POSTURES, MEDITATION, AND BREATHING EXERCISES... (SINGLE ISOLATED EXERCISES RECOMMENDED FOR USE DURING THE DAY ARE THE EXCEPTION)... DO NOT EAT OR DRINK FOR 1/2 HOUR AFTER PRACTICE. EMPTY BLADDER BEFORE PRACTICE.

## { BREATHING EXERCISES }

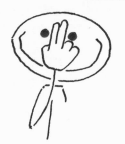 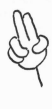 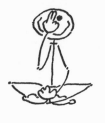

### BASIC HAND AND ARM POSITION

IN AN EASY POSE (P. 39), A THUNDERBOLT POSE (P. 40) OR SITTING ON A STRAIGHT CHAIR — KEEP SPINE ERECT, SHOULDERS RELAXED AND LEVEL, STERNUM PUSHED GENTLY FORWARD...

PLACE FIRST 2 FINGERS OF RIGHT HAND LIGHTLY ON CENTER OF FOREHEAD...REST TIP OF CURVED RIGHT THUMB ON RIGHT NOSTRIL (JUST ABOVE FLARE)...REST TIP OF CURVED RIGHT RING FINGER ON LEFT NOSTRIL (JUST ABOVE FLARE)... NEVER LIFT THUMB OR RING FINGER OFF NOSE (EITHER THE THUMBTIP AND/OR THE FINGERTIP VERY GENTLY SEALS A NOSTRIL, OR IT RESTS DELICATELY IN PLACE ON A NOSTRIL)...HOLD RIGHT WRIST FORWARD AWAY FROM MOUTH TO AVOID BREATHING DIRECTLY INTO PALM...REST RIGHT ARM AND ELBOW AGAINST SIDE.

### SUNBREATH

IN AN EASY POSE (P. 39), A THUNDERBOLT POSE (P. 40) OR SITTING ON A STRAIGHT CHAIR... BRING RIGHT HAND TO FACE IN BASIC HAND POSITION (ABOVE)...GENTLY SEAL LEFT NOSTRIL WITH RING FINGER...REST TIP OF THUMB ON RIGHT NOSTRIL (LEAVE RIGHT NOSTRIL OPEN)...CLOSE EYES...INHALE AND EXHALE DEEPLY, QUIETLY THROUGH RIGHT NOSTRIL (USING THE COMPLETE BREATH, P. 48 ).

## MID-CHEST BREATH

IN AN EASY POSE (P. 39 )
SPREAD FINGERS AND PLACE
PALMS ON RIBS JUST UNDER
SHOULDERS (FINGERS
POINTING TOWARD STERNUM
AND THUMBS AROUND BEHIND
BACK, UNDER SHOULDERBLADES)... KEEP
ABDOMINAL WALL QUIET... INHALE SLOWLY
THROUGH NOSE TO COMFORTABLY FILL
CHEST... FEEL RIBS EXPAND AGAINST PALMS,
FINGERS AND THUMBS... EXHALE AND
GENTLY SQUEEZE HANDS AGAINST RIBS
TO SLOWLY EMPTY LUNGS.

------------------------------------------------

## ABDOMINAL BREATH

IN AN EASY POSE (P. 39 )
SPREAD FINGERS AND PLACE
HANDS ON ABDOMINAL WALL
BETWEEN NAVEL AND PUBIS...
KEEP RIBCAGE QUIET AND
BREATHE SLOWLY IN AND OUT
THROUGH NOSE DURING ENTIRE EXERCISE...
INHALE AND EXHALE SLOWLY, QUIETLY TO
COMFORTABLY EXPAND AND FLATTEN
ABDOMINAL WALL... DO NOT FORCE
EXPANSION OF THE ABDOMINAL BALLOON.

------------------------------------------------

## SURFACE BREATH

IN A SPONGE POSE (P. 41)... CLOSE EYES...
RELAX ABDOMINAL WALL... BREATHE SLOWLY,
DEEPLY... IMAGINE AIR BEING
DRAWN IN AND RELEASED
THROUGH PORES...
"BREATHE" THROUGH
SKIN OVER ENTIRE
SURFACE OF BODY.

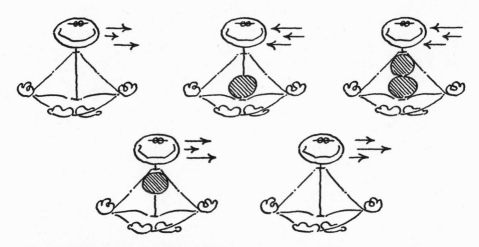

## COMPLETE BREATH

IN AN EASY POSE (P. 39), A SUPINE POSE (P. 40),
A SPONGE POSE (P. 41), A STANDING POSE
(P. 38) OR ON A STRAIGHT CHAIR...

IMAGINE THAT THERE ARE 2 BALLOONS
WITHIN THE TORSO – 1 WITHIN THE CHEST
AND 1 WITHIN THE ABDOMINAL CAVITY...
BREATHE SLOWLY AND QUIETLY THROUGH
NOSE DURING ENTIRE CYCLE...

TO INHALE: GENTLY FILL AND EXPAND THE
ABDOMINAL BALLOON WITH INCOMING AIR...
WHEN THE LOWER BALLOON IS COMFORTABLY
FULL, CONTINUE THE INHALATION TO FILL
THE CHEST BALLOON...

TO EXHALE: GENTLY TIGHTEN ABDOMINAL
WALL TO EMPTY ABDOMINAL BALLOON...
RELAX AND COLLAPSE RIBCAGE TO EMPTY
CHEST BALLOON...

BEGIN NEXT CYCLE IMMEDIATELY...

(THE COMPLETE BREATH IS RHYTHMIC,
EVEN AND QUIET).

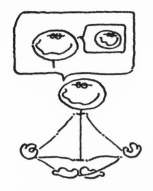

## MASTER BREATH

IN AN EASY POSE (P. 39), A SPONGE POSE (P. 41), OR SITTING ON A STRAIGHT CHAIR... CLOSE EYES... BREATHE QUIETLY AND NATURALLY... CAREFULLY <u>OBSERVE</u> FLOW OF AIR <u>WITHOUT INTERFERING WITH BREATHING PATTERN</u> IN ANY WAY.

---

## ALTERNATE NOSTRIL BREATH

IN AN EASY POSE (P. 39), A THUNDERBOLT POSE (P. 40), OR SITTING ON A STRAIGHT CHAIR... BRING RIGHT HAND TO FACE IN BASIC HAND POSITION (P. 46)... USE A SMOOTH, QUIET, RHYTHMIC COMPLETE BREATH (P. 48) DURING ENTIRE EXERCISE...

(GENTLY SEAL LEFT NOSTRIL)... <u>INHALE</u> SLOWLY THROUGH <u>RIGHT</u> NOSTRIL... (SEAL RIGHT NOSTRIL AND OPEN LEFT)... <u>EXHALE</u> THROUGH <u>LEFT</u> NOSTRIL... <u>INHALE</u> THROUGH <u>LEFT</u> NOSTRIL... (SEAL LEFT NOSTRIL AND OPEN RIGHT)... <u>EXHALE</u> THROUGH <u>RIGHT</u> NOSTRIL... (THIS COMPLETES 1 BREATH CYCLE)... BEGIN AGAIN.

BREATHE –
IN RIGHT, OUT LEFT
IN LEFT, OUT RIGHT
IN RIGHT, OUT LEFT
IN LEFT, OUT RIGHT.....

R.                L.

---

## CALM BREATH

CALM
CAAALM
CAAAALM

IN AN EASY POSE (P. 39) OR ON A STRAIGHT CHAIR... CLOSE EYES... RELAX FACE AND SHOULDER MUSCLES... BREATHE DEEPLY, USING A COMPLETE BREATH (P. 48)... DURING EACH EXHALATION SILENTLY REPEAT THE WORD "CALM".

## RHYTHMIC BREATH

IN AN EASY POSE (P. 39), A
SUPINE POSE (P. 40), A SPONGE
POSE (P. 41) OR ON A
STRAIGHT CHAIR...CLOSE
EYES...RELAX ABDOMEN...
INHALE SLOWLY THROUGH
NOSE, COUNTING NUMBER OF
SECONDS NECESSARY TO FILL LUNGS
COMFORTABLY...USE SAME NUMBER OF
SECONDS TO HOLD BREATH, TO EXHALE,
TO REMAIN EMPTY (THE RATIO OF IN-HOLD-
OUT-HOLD IS 1:1:1:1)...BEGIN CYCLE AGAIN.

1:1:1:1

---

## MOON BREATH

IN AN EASY POSE (P. 39), A THUNDERBOLT
POSE (P. 40), OR SITTING ON A STRAIGHT
CHAIR...BRING RIGHT HAND
TO FACE IN BASIC HAND
POSITION (P. 46)...GENTLY SEAL
RIGHT NOSTRIL WITH TIP OF THUMB...
REST TIP OF RING FINGER ON LEFT NOSTRIL
(LEAVE LEFT NOSTRIL OPEN)...CLOSE
EYES... INHALE AND EXHALE DEEPLY,
QUIETLY THROUGH LEFT NOSTRIL (USING
THE COMPLETE BREATH, P. 48).

---

## PERFECT BREATH

IN A SPONGE POSE (P. 41)...BREATHE QUIETLY
THROUGH NOSE, USING A COMPLETE BREATH
(P. 48)...INHALE SLOWLY, COUNTING NUMBER
OF SECONDS NECESSARY TO COMFORTABLY
FILL LUNGS...DOUBLE THAT TIME FOR
EXHALATION, USING
A 1:2 RATIO...
DURING EACH
EXHALATION IMAGINE
ALL MENTAL AND
PHYSICAL TENSION
FLOATING AWAY WITH
OUTGOING AIR.

## SIPPING BREATH

IN AN EASY POSE (P. 39), A THUNDERBOLT POSE
(P. 40), OR SITTING ON A STRAIGHT CHAIR....
STICK TONGUE OUT ABOUT 1 INCH BEYOND
LIPS... SHAPE MOUTH INTO AN "O" TO CURL
TONGUE INTO A SOFT, NARROW
TUBE (GROVE WILL BE ON TOP
OF TONGUE)... INHALE SLOWLY
THROUGH TUBE, USING A
COMPLETE BREATH (P. 48 )...
WHEN LUNGS ARE FULL, BRING
TONGUE IN AND CLOSE MOUTH...
EXHALE THROUGH NOSE...BEGIN AGAIN.

---

## COMFORTABLE BREATH

IN AN EASY POSE (P. 39) OR ON A STRAIGHT
CHAIR....CLOSE EYES...RELAX ABDOMEN...
INHALE SLOWLY THROUGH NOSE, COUNTING
NUMBER OF SECONDS NECESSARY TO FILL
LUNGS COMFORTABLY... HOLD
BREATH 4 TIMES AS LONG AS
LENGTH OF INHALATION...
EXHALE, TAKING 2 TIMES
AS LONG AS INHALATION...
(RATIO OF IN-HOLD-OUT IS
1:4:2)...BEGIN AGAIN.

1:4:2

---

## FLOWING BREATH

FROM AN EASY POSE (P. 39), A THUNDERBOLT
POSE (P. 40), OR SITTING ON A STRAIGHT CHAIR..
CLOSE EYES... INHALE SLOWLY, USING A
COMPLETE BREATH (P. 48)...DURING EACH
INHALATION IMAGINE THAT A BEAUTIFUL
FLOW OF HEALING, REFRESHING ENERGY
ENTERS BASE OF SPINE AND RISES UP
SPINAL COLUMN TO HEAD...

DURING EACH EXHALATION
IMAGINE THAT FLOW OF
ENERGY RADIATES AND
SHINES OUTWARD FROM
CENTER OF FOREHEAD...
BEGIN AGAIN.

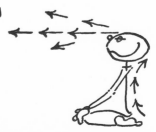

# DEEP RELAXATION

THERE FLOWS THROUGH EACH OF US A CURRENT OF COSMIC ENERY - ENERGY THAT HEALS, STRENGTHENS, CLEANSES, NOURISHES... THIS ENERGY IS OUR BIRTHRIGHT, AND IT IS GIVEN LOVINGLY... IT IS GIVEN WITHOUT QUALIFICATION OR HESITATION... IF YOU HOPE TO REALIZE YOUR FULL POTENTIAL, YOU MUST ALLOW THIS CURRENT TO FLOW AS FREELY AS A MOUNTAIN STREAM THROUGH MIND, BODY, AND SPIRIT... TENSION "DAMS" CAUSE THE ENERGY TO STAGNATE - OR THE "DAMS" MAY EVENTUALLY BURST, DESTROYING A PART OF THE PHYSICAL OR MENTAL MACHINERY... SPEND AT LEAST A FEW MOMENTS EACH DAY UNWINDING, LETTING GO... PRACTICE THE ART OF RELAXATION AS OFTEN AS POSSIBLE...

1. FROM A SPONGE POSE (P. 41), EASY POSE (P.39), OR ON A STRAIGHT CHAIR.... CLOSE EYES...
2. RELAX SKIN TENSION (IMAGINE SKIN OF SCALP, FACE AND BODY IS WARM, LOOSE SOFT)...
3. IMAGINE THE EYELIDS BECOMING HEAVY...
4. LET GO OF, "DISCONNECT", THE TOES, ANKLES, CALVES, KNEES, THIGHS, LOWER SPINE, BUTTOCKS, ABDOMINAL WALL, SHOULDERBLADES, SHOULDERS, ARMS, WRISTS, FINGERS, BACK OF NECK, THROAT, JAWS, TONGUE, MUSCLES THAT CIRCLE THE MOUTH AND EYES, FOREHEAD AND SCALP...
5. IMAGINE THE BONES ARE AS LIGHT AS A SPARROW'S...
6. "GIVE IN" TO GRAVITY'S DOWNWARD PULL.

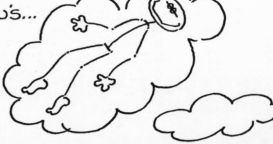

# PASSIVE meditation

YOU ARE A GOD IN THE MAKING...

YOUR <u>TOTAL</u> <u>SELF</u> IS THE ARCHITECT RESPONSIBLE FOR YOUR UNFOLDING, FOR YOUR BECOMING... YOUR <u>TOTAL</u> <u>SELF</u> HAS ACCESS TO AN UNLIMITED SUPPLY OF COSMIC BUILDING MATERIALS – PATIENCE, STRENGTH, COURAGE...THERE IS WITHIN YOUR <u>TOTAL</u> <u>SELF</u> THE KNOWINGNESS OF WHO AND WHY YOU ARE, OF WHERE YOU HAVE BEEN AND WHERE YOU ARE GOING... YOUR <u>TOTAL</u> <u>SELF</u> UNDERSTANDS THAT YOU ARE AN INDESTRUCTIBLE AND INDISPENSABLE PORTION OF THE COSMOS...

AS THE <u>TOTAL</u> <u>SELF</u> IS A PART OF THE COSMOS, THE <u>FRACTIONAL</u> <u>SELF</u> IS A SMALLER PORTION OF THE <u>TOTAL</u> <u>SELF</u>... YOUR <u>FRACTIONAL</u> <u>SELF</u> IS A SPECIAL COMBINATION OF TRAITS AND ABILITIES THAT ENABLES YOU TO FOCUS CLEARLY AND TO FUNCTION SMOOTHLY WITHIN OUR TEMPORARY PHYSICAL ENVIRONMENT... WHEN YOU ASSUME THAT YOUR <u>FRACTIONAL</u> <u>SELF</u> IS YOUR <u>TOTAL</u> <u>SELF</u>, YOU ARE FORCING THE LIMITED SPECIALIZED <u>FRACTIONAL</u> <u>SELF</u> TO PERFORM COSMIC-LEVEL DUTIES FOR WHICH IT'S NOT DESIGNED...

IF YOU ASSUME THAT YOUR <u>FRACTIONAL</u> <u>SELF</u> IS YOUR HIGHEST SOURCE, YOU MAY ALSO LOSE SIGHT OF YOUR COSMIC HERITAGE, YOUR COSMIC GROWTH AND YOUR COSMIC POWER....

DECISIONS MADE AND COURSES CHARTED FOR YOU BY YOUR TOTAL SELF WILL ALWAYS INCLUDE WHAT IS BEST FOR YOUR FRACTIONAL SELF... DECISIONS MADE BY THE FRACTIONAL SELF ARE OFTEN MYOPIC AND MAY NOT REPRESENT WHAT IS BEST FOR YOUR TOTAL SELF... TO DENY ONE'S TOTAL SELF IS TO LEAD A RESTRICTED, RESTLESS LIFE, OFTEN A WASTED LIFE...

PASSIVE MEDITATION IS RESTING QUIETLY, LISTENING TO - BEING AWARE OF - THE TOTAL YOU... LET PASSIVE MEDITATION BECOME AN IMPORTANT AND CHERISHED PART OF EVERY DAY... TO DO WITHOUT IT IS LIKE TRYING TO PLAY CHOPIN ON A KAZOO...

THE INTENT TO REACH OUT TO YOUR TOTAL SELF IS FAR MORE IMPORTANT THAN THE MEDITATIVE RITUAL OR TECHNIQUE... THE FOLLOWING FORMULA IS ONLY A SEED, A SMALL BEGINNING (LATER, YOUR TOTAL SELF MAY REPLACE THIS FORMULA WITH ONE MORE SUITABLE FOR YOUR OWN TEMPERMENT AND LIFESTYLE)...

1. PRACTICE DEEP RELAXATION (P. 52) UNTIL THE BODY IS COMFORTABLE AND QUIET...

2. PRACTICE THE ABDOMINAL BREATH (P. 47) OR THE PERFECT BREATH (P. 50) UNTIL THE BREATH FLOWS EASILY, QUIETLY...

3. RESUME NATURAL BREATHING... SILENTLY "EXHALE" THE WORD "ONE" WITH EACH BREATH CYCLE... IMAGINE THE WORD FLOATING OUT OF THE BODY AND DRIFTING FAR OUT INTO THE COSMOS... (ALLOW THE THOUGHT-FRAGMENTS TO FLOAT UNDISTURBED BY THE MIND'S EYE AND THE MIND WILL CLEAR QUICKLY)... TRY TO ALLOW AT LEAST 10 MINUTES FOR STEP 3.

# CREATIVE MEDITATION

THE PRACTICE OF PASSIVE MEDITATION (P. 53) EXPANDS AND EXTENDS YOUR AWARENESS TO INCLUDE YOUR CREATIVE, SERENE TOTAL SELF... YOUR TOTAL SELF IS AN ARTIST DEDICATED TO YOUR UNFOLDING... THE SHAPING AND POLISHING OF YOUR OWN MIND-BODY-SPIRIT IS THE PERFECTING OF ONE PIECE OF THE LARGER, EXPANDING MOSAIC OF THE COSMOS... THE TOTAL MOSAIC IS STRENGTHENED AND REFINED BECAUSE OF YOUR OWN INDIVIDUAL EFFORTS ... DURING CREATIVE MEDITATION THE TOTAL SELF IS GIVEN SPECIFIC CREATIVE WORK TO DO:

1. SELECT, AND CLEARLY VERBALIZE, A TRAIT YOU BELIEVE YOU NEED FOR YOUR COSMIC GROWTH (PERHAPS A STRONG BODY TO EXPLORE THE OUTER ENVIRONMENT, OR PERHAPS A CALM MIND TO EXPLORE YOUR INNER ENVIRONMENT)...
2. COMPLETE THE 3 STEPS OF PASSIVE MEDITATION (P. 53)...
3. BREATHE NATURALLY... IMAGINE THAT THE INBREATH BRINGS WITH IT POWERFUL, RADIANT ENERGY... SILENTLY REPEAT THE SELECTED PHRASE DURING THE OUTBREATH (INFUSING THE PHRASE WITH ENERGY)... TRY TO ALLOW AT LEAST 10 MINUTES FOR THIS STEP...
4. AS IF WATCHING A FILM, PICTURE YOURSELF FUNCTIONING WITH AN ABUNDANCE OF THE QUALITY YOU NEED...

EVERY CREATION BEGINS WITH AN IDEA - A BLUEPRINT... WE ARE OFTEN SHAPED BY OLD BLUEPRINTS WHICH INHIBIT OUR GROWTH... YOU, AS TOTAL SELF, HAVE THE POWER TO REPLACE, TO REDESIGN, THOSE BLUEPRINTS THROUGH CREATIVE MEDITATION.

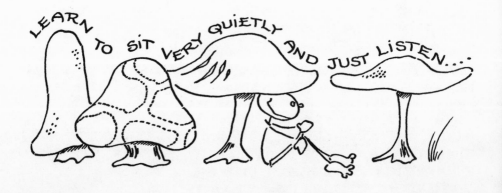

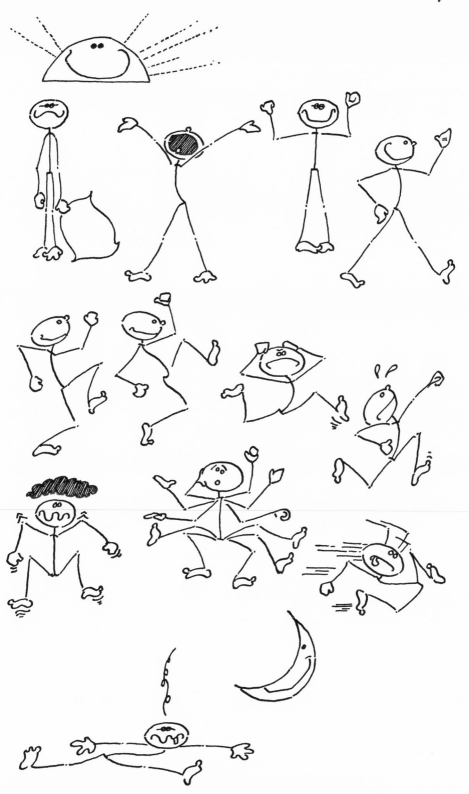

THE FOLLOWING SUGGESTIONS ARE OFFERED AS "YOGIC TOOLS"-TOOLS TO BE USED IN YOUR DAILY LIFE... THIS SECTION IS NOT MEANT TO PROVIDE A RIGID FORMULA - IT IS ONLY A REMINDER OF YOUR OWN CREATIVITY AS AN ARTIST INVOLVED IN THE SHAPING OF YOURSELF.

## INSOMNIA

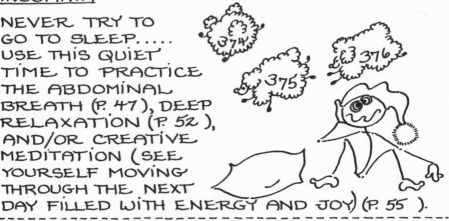

NEVER TRY TO GO TO SLEEP..... USE THIS QUIET TIME TO PRACTICE THE ABDOMINAL BREATH (P. 47), DEEP RELAXATION (P. 52), AND/OR CREATIVE MEDITATION (SEE YOURSELF MOVING THROUGH THE NEXT DAY FILLED WITH ENERGY AND JOY) (P. 55).

## ANGER

ANGER IS OFTEN CAUSED BY THE NARROW LIMITED VISION OF THE FRACTIONAL SELF...PRACTICE PASSIVE MEDITATION DAILY (P. 53)... DURING DIFFICULT TIMES PRACTICE THE COMPLETE BREATH (P. 48) OR THE CALM BREATH (P. 49).

## HEADACHE

DEEP RELAXATION WITH SPECIAL EMPHASIS ON MUSCLES OF FACE, NECK, SHOULDERS (P. 52)... HEAD TILT (P. 72)...NECK ROLL (P.122).. SHOULDER LIFT (P.83)... FLOWING BREATH (P. 51)... ALTERNATE NOSTRIL BREATH (P. 49)...IF PAIN PERSISTS, CHECK WITH YOUR DOCTOR.

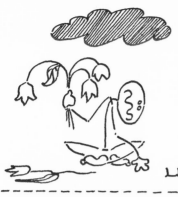

### DEPRESSION

TRY THE SUNBREATH (P. 46), OR COMPLETE BREATH (P. 48)... USE STEP 4 OF CREATIVE MEDITATION (P. 55) TO IMAGINE THAT YOUR HEART IS A SMALL SUN WITHIN YOU - THE "SUN" RADIATES WARMTH AND LIGHT THROUGH YOUR BEING.

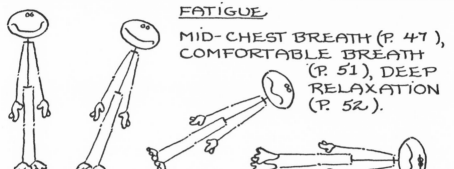

### FATIGUE

MID-CHEST BREATH (P. 47), COMFORTABLE BREATH (P. 51), DEEP RELAXATION (P. 52).

### PAIN

THROUGH THE DAILY PRACTICE OF PASSIVE AND CREATIVE MEDITATION (PP 55) YOU WILL LEARN THAT PAIN CAN BE ONLY A TINY PART OF YOUR FRACTIONAL SELF... TRY 1-POINT CONCENTRATION, DEEP RELAXATION (P. 52), RHYTHMIC BREATH (P. 50).

### PHOBIAS AND FEARS

USE STEP 4 OF CREATIVE MEDITATION (P. 55) TO PICTURE YOURSELF (RADIANT AND CALM) HELPING OTHERS OVERCOME THESE SAME FEARS... IN TIMES OF STRESS TRY THE CALM BREATH (P. 49) OR THE ABDOMINAL BREATH (P. 47)... REMEMBER THAT TOTAL SELF IS NOT AFRAID.

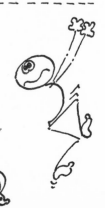

### SHYNESS

IS A FRACTIONAL SELF-ISHNESS. IF YOU ARE SHY, YOU ARE TRYING TO FUNCTION WHILE IN A FETAL POSITION. SUGGESTION: GET ACQUAINTED WITH YOUR TOTAL SELF THROUGH PASSIVE MEDITATION (P. 53). USE STEP 4 OF CREATIVE MEDITATION TO PICTURE YOURSELF COUNSELING OTHERS WHO ARE SHY. (P. 55).

---

### POOR CIRCULATION

GIVE SPECIAL ATTENTION TO: SALUTATION TO THE SUN (P. 150), SALUTATION TO THE MOON (P. 153), FORWARD STRETCHING BREATH (P. 71), COMFORTABLE BREATH (P. 51), AND THE MINI-POSES (PP 63-67).

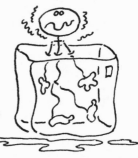

---

### TENSION

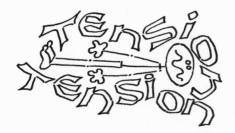

TRY: PERFECT BREATH (P. 50), CALM BREATH (P. 49), ALTERNATE NOSTRIL BREATH (P. 49), ABDOMINAL BREATH (P. 47) AND/OR DEEP RELAXATION (P. 52).

---

### A TRAPPED FEELING

TRY THE TEMPLE BREATH (P. 72) OR THE COMPLETE BREATH (P. 48)... IF THERE IS TIME, CREATE YOUR OWN SALUTATION... USE STEP 4 OF CREATIVE MEDITATION (P. 55) TO SET YOUR MIND FREE TO "EXPLORE" (INNER CHAMBERS OF A SEASHELL, DARK SIDE OF THE MOON, AN EAGLE'S NEST, THE HEART OF A REDWOOD.....).

## OVEREATING

IS A FRACTIONAL-SELF HABIT— AN OLD
DESTRUCTIVE BLUEPRINT....PRACTICE
PASSIVE MEDITATION (P. 53) DAILY...USE
CREATIVE MEDITATION (P. 55) TO DESIGN
IN YOUR MIND A NEW YOU— LEAN, STRONG,
CALM.... SUBSTITUTE A BREATHING-BREAK
FOR A COFFEE-BREAK...PRACTICE DEEP
RELAXATION BEFORE EVENING MEALS
(P. 52).....FORGET DIETING — PROPER
NOURISHMENT OF THE MIND-BODY-SPIRIT
IS AN ONGOING CREATIVE EFFORT....IT
IS A PLUS, NOT A MINUS.... CROWD OUT OLD
HABITS WITH NEW ONES.

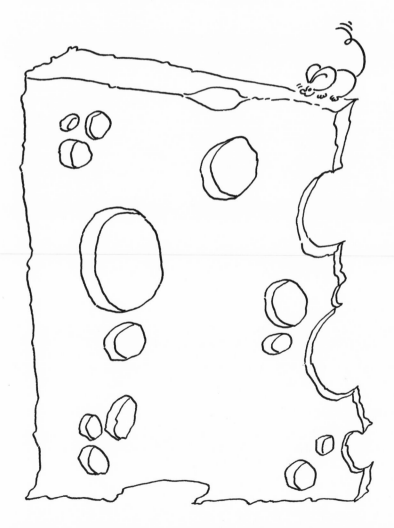

## LONG TRIPS

MINI-POSES (PP 63-67)...
DEEP RELAXATION
(P. 52 )... COMFORTABLE
BREATH (P. 51 )...
RHYTHMIC BREATH (P. 50 )...
FLOWING BREATH (P. 51 ).

MOVE AND WIGGLE
AS MUCH AS POSSIBLE.

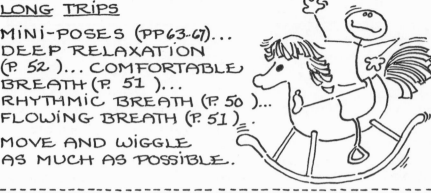

- - - - - - - - - - - - - - - - - - - - - - - - - - - -

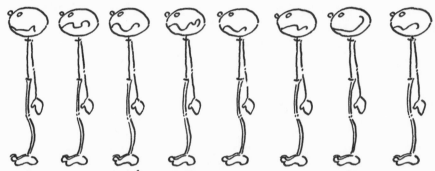

## LOOOOOONG LINES AND OTHER TEDIUM

CLOCK (P. 75 )... RHYTHMIC BREATH (P. 50 )...
COMFORTABLE BREATH (P. 51 ).... OR,
BREATHE NATURALLY AND REPEAT
SILENTLY "MY BODY IS STRONG" (DURING
INBREATH) - "MY MIND IS AT PEACE" (DURING
OUTBREATH).

- - - - - - - - - - - - - - - - - - - - - - - - - - - -

## EXAMS, CONFERENCES, INTERVIEWS....

NIGHT BEFORE : PRACTICE CREATIVE
MEDITATION (P. 55 ) - VISUALIZE YOURSELF
COMPLETING THE TASK, CALMLY AND
CONFIDENTLY...... BEFORE EXAM: TRY
ALTERNATE NOSTRIL BREATH
(P. 49 )..... DURING EXAM:
ABDOMINAL BREATH (P. 47),
AND COMPLETE BREATH
(P. 48 )...THINK ONLY OF
THE QUALITY OF YOUR
WORK - NEVER OF
THE RESULTS.

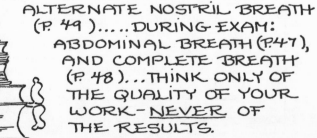

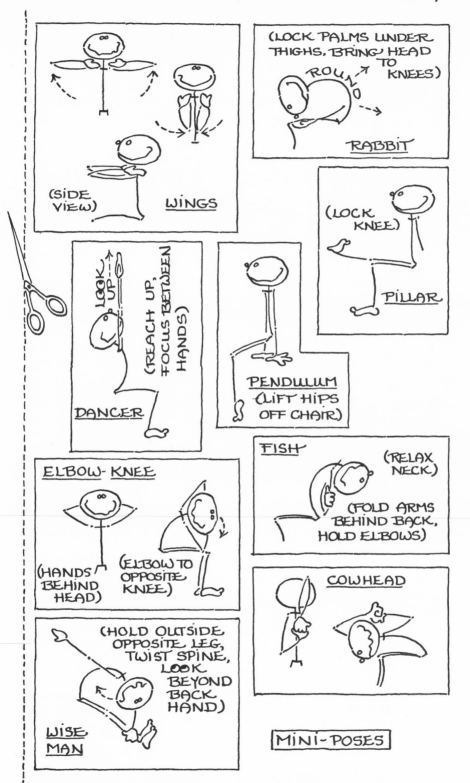

(SIDE VIEW)    WINGS

(LOCK PALMS UNDER THIGHS, BRING HEAD TO KNEES)
ROUND
RABBIT

(LOCK KNEE)
PILLAR

LOOK UP
(REACH UP, FOCUS BETWEEN HANDS)
DANCER

PENDULUM
(LIFT HIPS OFF CHAIR)

FISH
(RELAX NECK)
(FOLD ARMS BEHIND BACK, HOLD ELBOWS)

ELBOW-KNEE
(HANDS BEHIND HEAD)
(ELBOW TO OPPOSITE KNEE)

COWHEAD

(HOLD OUTSIDE OPPOSITE LEG, TWIST SPINE, LOOK BEYOND BACK HAND)
WISE MAN

MINI-POSES

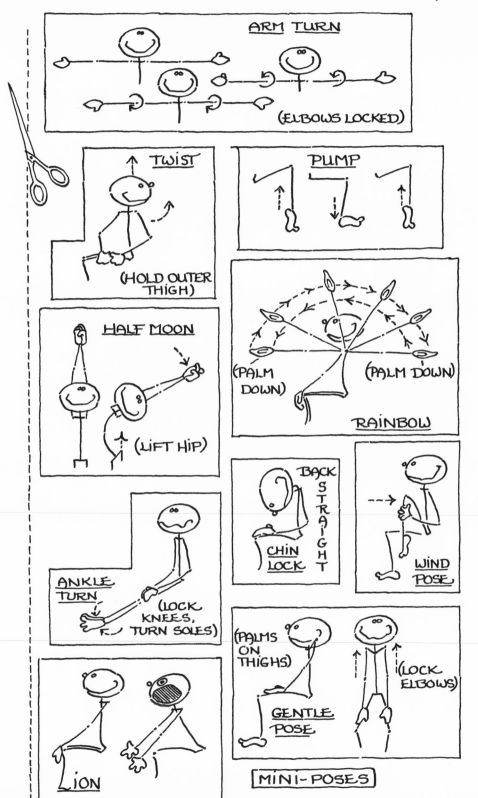

ARM TURN

(ELBOWS LOCKED)

TWIST

(HOLD OUTER THIGH)

PUMP

HALF MOON

(LIFT HIP)

(PALM DOWN)     (PALM DOWN)

RAINBOW

BACK STRAIGHT

CHIN LOCK

WIND POSE

ANKLE TURN

(LOCK KNEES, TURN SOLES)

(PALMS ON THIGHS)

GENTLE POSE

(LOCK ELBOWS)

LION

MINI-POSES

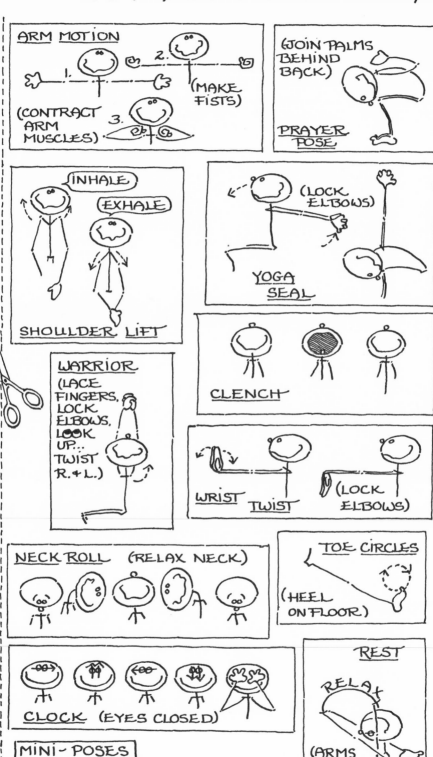

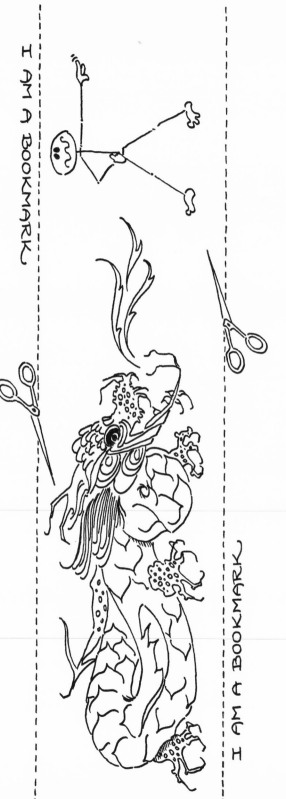

I AM A BOOKMARK

I AM A BOOKMARK

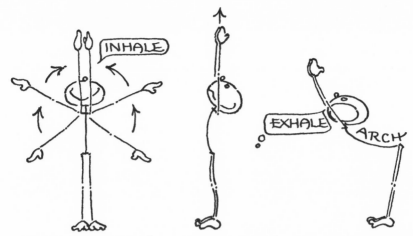

1. FROM A STANDING POSE (P. 38) SEPARATE FEET HIP-WIDTH APART...RELAX ABDOMINAL WALL... INHALE SLOWLY THROUGH NOSE WHILE STRETCHING ARMS OUT SIDEWAYS AND UP OVER HEAD (HANDS SHOULDER-WIDTH APART)...FOCUS BETWEEN HANDS... ARCH SPINE BACKWARD...

2. OPEN MOUTH-THROAT WIDE AS IF TO YAWN... EXHALE EVENLY AND DEEPLY WHILE REACHING FORWARD AND DOWN (MOUTH REMAINS OPEN WIDE FOR ENTIRE EXHALATION)..

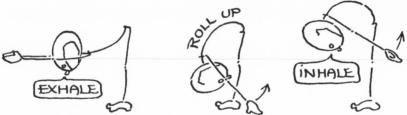

3. AT THE END OF EXHALATION RELAX ARMS, NECK, AND ABDOMINAL WALL... INHALE AGAIN SLOWLY THROUGH NOSE WHILE STRETCHING ARMS OUT SIDEWAYS AND UP...REPEAT CYCLE BY INHALING WHILE TRACING A CIRCLE FROM FLOOR TO CEILING, BY EXHALING WHILE SLICING THAT CIRCLE IN HALF...MOVEMENT AND BREATH SHOULD BE EVEN AND SMOOTH.

{STRETCHING BREATH, FORWARD}

## {TEMPLE BREATH}

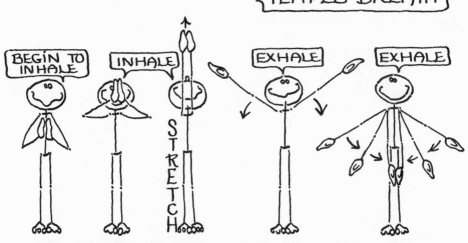

1. FROM A STANDING POSE (P. 38 ) SEPARATE FEET 1 INCH APART...BREATHE DEEPLY-QUIETLY THROUGH NOSE DURING ENTIRE EXERCISE... (MOVEMENT SHOULD BE CONSTANT AND GRACEFUL)...JOIN PALMS IN FRONT OF CHEST... RELAX ABDOMINAL WALL DURING EACH INHALATION...

2. <u>INHALE</u> SLOWLY WHILE: MOVING JOINED HANDS IN FRONT OF FACE AND STRAIGHT UP AS FAR AS POSSIBLE...(LUNGS SHOULD BE COMFORTABLY FULL AT THIS POINT)...

3. <u>EXHALE</u> SLOWLY AND COMPLETELY WHILE: SWEEPING ARMS OUT SIDEWAYS, THEN DOWN TO JOIN PALMS AGAIN... CONTINUE TO BREATHE <u>OUT</u> AS HANDS MOVE UP TO CHEST LEVEL...

4. RELAX ABDOMEN AND BEGIN AGAIN...

- - - - - - - - - - - - - - - - - - - - - - - - - - - - - - - - - -

## {HEAD TILT 2}

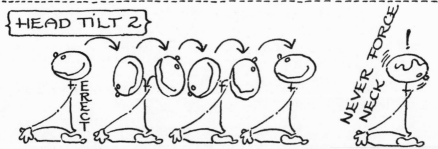

KEEP BACK ERECT AND STERNUM LIFTED...RELAX NECK... SLOWLY-SMOOTHLY TILT HEAD FORWARD AND BACKWARD...ALLOW WEIGHT OF HEAD TO STRETCH NECK.

{HAND TO FOOT 1}

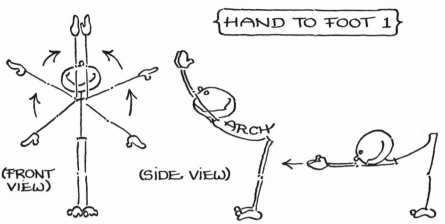

(FRONT VIEW)   (SIDE VIEW)

1. FROM A STANDING POSE (P. 38) SEPARATE FEET HIP-WIDTH APART... STRETCH ARMS SIDEWAYS AND UP OVER HEAD... LIFT CHIN (FOCUS BEYOND HANDS DURING FORWARD STRETCH)...

2. ARCH SPINE GENTLY BACKWARD... LOCK KNEES... STRETCH AND REACH AS FAR <u>FORWARD</u> AS POSSIBLE, THEN AS FAR <u>DOWN</u> AS POSSIBLE...

3. STRETCH FROM COCCYX ⟶ FINGERTIPS ⟶

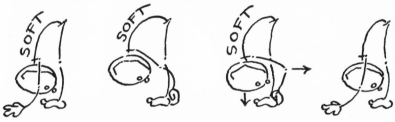

4. <u>DEEPLY</u> <u>RELAX</u> <u>NECK</u>, <u>SHOULDERS</u>, FULL LENGTH OF <u>SPINE</u>, <u>ABDOMINAL</u> <u>WALL</u> (KEEP THESE AREAS SOFT!)... FOCUS ON REAR WALL...

5. PINCH EACH ACHILLES TENDON BETWEEN THUMB AND FINGERS...

6. BEND ELBOWS STEADILY BACKWARD... KEEP NECK AND ABDOMEN SOFT... [HOLD]...

7. RELEASE HEELS... PAUSE... STRETCH SLOWLY FORWARD AND UP TO CEILING... FLOAT ARMS OUT SIDEWAYS AND DOWN TO OUTER THIGHS... REST IN A STANDING POSE.

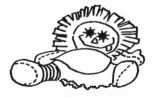

## {HEAD TO KNEE 3}

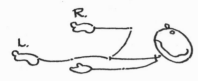

1. FROM A SUPINE POSE (P. 40) DRAW BENT RIGHT KNEE TOWARD CHEST... KEEP RIGHT SHIN LEVEL...

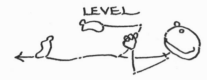

2. INTERLOCK FINGERS BEHIND THIGH (HALFWAY BETWEEN KNEE AND HIP) ..PUSH LEFT HEEL AWAY FROM BODY...

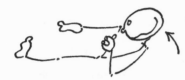

3. SLOWLY RAISE HEAD...KEEP SHOULDERS PULLED AWAY FROM NECK, ARMS CLOSE TO BODY...TOUCH FACE ON KNEE... HOLD ...

4. "FLOAT" HEAD DOWN TO FLOOR...RELEASE AND EXTEND RIGHT LEG...LOWER ARMS...REPEAT POSE (OTHER SIDE) BRINGING LEFT KNEE TO CHEST...REST IN A SUPINE POSE.

-----------------------------------------------

## {SHOULDER SHIFT}

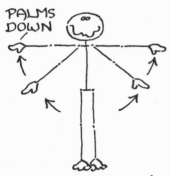

PALMS DOWN

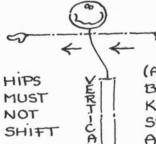

HIPS MUST NOT SHIFT

VERTICAL

(AT FIRST IT MAY BE HELPFUL TO KEEP HIPS AND SHOULDERS AGAINST A WALL)

1. FROM A STANDING POSE (P. 38) SEPARATE FEET HIP-WIDTH APART...STRETCH ARMS SIDEWAYS AT SHOULDER LEVEL...KEEP HIPS-LEGS EXACTLY IN PLACE, SHOULDERS DOWN-LEVEL, NECK LONG-STRAIGHT AND ARMS GENTLY STRETCHED...
2. SHIFT RIBCAGE AS FAR RIGHT AS POSSIBLE (AS IF SLIDING ACROSS A WALL)...FOCUS STRAIGHT AHEAD... HOLD
3. STRAIGHTEN SPINE...REPEAT POSE, SHIFTING AND SLIDING CHEST LEFT...REST IN A STANDING POSE.

{TRIANGLE 1}

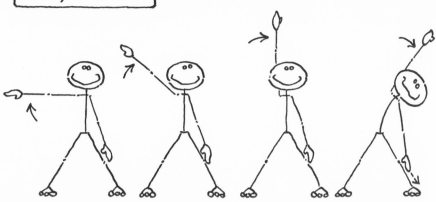

1. FROM A SPREAD FOOT POSE (P. 39) SEPARATE FEET
3 FEET APART... KEEP INNER EDGES OF FEET
PARALLEL, KNEES LOCKED... IN 1 FLOWING MOTION
STRETCH RIGHT ARM OUT SIDEWAYS AND UP OVER
HEAD... TURN RIGHT PALM LEFT... SLOWLY SLIDE
LEFT PALM DOWN OUTSIDE LEFT LEG AS FAR AS
POSSIBLE... KEEP RIGHT ARM NEAR RIGHT EAR...

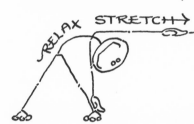

2. KEEP BOTH SHOULDERS SAME
DISTANCE FROM FRONT WALL
(MOVE AS IF BACK IS FLAT
AGAINST REAR WALL)...
KEEP RIGHT ARM STRAIGHT,
LEVEL WITH FLOOR AND IN
LINE WITH LEFT ANKLEBONE..
RELAX NECK... FOCUS STRAIGHT AHEAD... STRETCH
RIGHT ARM GENTLY... RELAX RIGHT SIDE... [HOLD]..

3 ROLL UP SLOWLY (RIGHT ARM AND HEAD TOGETHER)..
BRING RIGHT ARM DOWN TO OUTER RIGHT THIGH...
REPEAT POSE (OTHER SIDE), STRETCHING LEFT ARM
OVER HEAD... REST IN STANDING POSE (P. 38).

- - - - - - - - - - - - - - - - - - - - - - - - - - - - - - - - - - - -

{CLOCK}

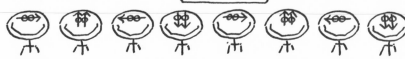

1. CLOSE EYES... ROLL EYES VERY SLOWLY,
AS IF READING NUMBERS ON A
GIANT CLOCK (REPEAT EXERCISE
CLOCKWISE AND COUNTERCLOCKWISE)...
2. GENTLY CUP PALMS OVER CLOSED EYES.. [HOLD].

## { WISE MAN POSE }

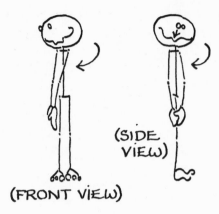

(SIDE VIEW)

(FRONT VIEW)

1. FROM A STANDING POSE (P. 38)... SEPARATE FEET HIP-DISTANCE APART... KEEP LEGS VERTICAL DURING POSE...LOCK KNEES... KEEP BOTH HIPBONES EXACTLY SAME DISTANCE FROM FRONT WALL...TURN UPPER BODY RIGHT...PLACE BOTH PALMS ON OUTER RIGHT HIP...

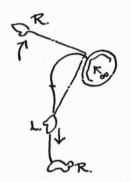 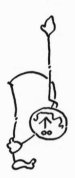 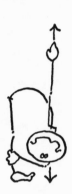

2. FOCUS BEYOND RAISED HAND... IN 1 FLOWING MOTION: TWIST AND LENGTHEN SPINE, SLIDE LEFT PALM DOWN OUTSIDE RIGHT LEG, STRETCH RIGHT ARM STRAIGHT BACK FROM OUTER RIGHT HIP AND THEN STRAIGHT UP...KEEP RIGHT PALM TURNED TOWARD BODY...

3. GRASP OUTER RIGHT CALF, ANKLE OR HEEL WITH LEFT HAND... DO NOT ALLOW HIPS TO PIVOT... FOCUS ON CEILING BEYOND RIGHT THUMB...

4. GENTLY BEND LEFT ELBOW TO BRING TOP OF HEAD CLOSER TO FLOOR ... STRETCH RIGHT ARM STRAIGHT UP... [HOLD] ...

5. SLOWLY STRAIGHTEN UP, SLIDING LEFT HAND UP RIGHT LEG AND LOWERING RIGHT ARM...FACE FORWARD...REPEAT POSE (OTHER SIDE), PLACING PALMS ON OUTER LEFT HIP... REST IN A STANDING POSE.

## { SMALL MOUNTAIN }

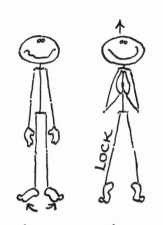

1. FROM A STANDING POSE (P.38) SEPARATE PARALLEL FEET HIP-DISTANCE APART...TURN TOES HALFWAY OUT (CREATE A RIGHT ANGLE BETWEEN INNER EDGES OF FEET)...
2. JOIN PALMS IN FRONT OF CHEST AND REST ELBOWS AGAINST SIDES...<u>STRETCH TOP OF HEAD TOWARD CEILING DURING POSE</u>...
RISE AS HIGH ON TOES AS POSSIBLE...(GENTLY PUSH FRONT OF FOOT OUT OVER TOES TO DEEPEN ARCH AND LOCK FOOT)...LOCK KNEES...FOCUS STRAIGHT AHEAD... HOLD ...
3. SLOWLY LOWER HEELS AND HANDS...TURN TOES FORWARD...REST IN A STANDING POSE.

-------------------------------------------------------

## { THIGH POSE }

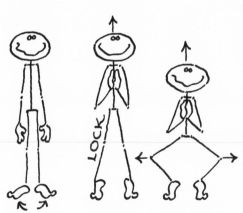

1. FROM A STANDING POSE (P.38) SEPARATE PARALLEL FEET HIP-DISTANCE APART... TURN TOES OUT CREATING A RIGHT ANGLE BETWEEN INNER EDGES OF FEET... <u>KEEP SPINE STRETCHED UP AND BACK ERECT</u>...
2. SLOWLY BEND KNEES <u>OUTWARD</u> (IN LINE WITH TOES), COMING AS HIGH ON TOES AS POSSIBLE...
3. FOCUS STRAIGHT AHEAD... LOWER BODY INTO A HALF SQUAT, KEEPING HEELS HIGH AND KNEES PUSHING OUTWARD... HOLD ...
4. STRAIGHTEN LEGS IN 1 SMOOTH MOVEMENT... LOWER HEELS AND HANDS...TURN TOES FORWARD...REST IN A STANDING POSE.

## {UNEVEN POSE}

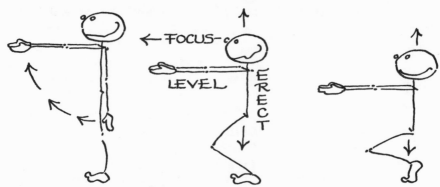

1. FROM A STANDING POSE (P. 38) SEPARATE
   PARALLEL FEET HIP-WIDTH APART... STRETCH
   BOTH ARMS FORWARD (SHOULDER-WIDTH APART,
   PALMS DOWN AND LEVEL WITH FLOOR.)...PRESS
   INNER KNEES AND INNER THIGHS FIRMLY
   TOGETHER...KEEP SPINE STRAIGHT...FOCUS...

2. GENTLY TUCK SEAT UNDER AND BEND KNEES...
   REACH TOWARD CEILING WITH TOP OF HEAD
   DURING ENTIRE POSE...RELAX SHOULDERS...

3. LOWER BODY INTO A FULL SQUAT, RISING UP ON
   TOES ON THE WAY DOWN (KNEES TOGETHER)...

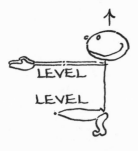

4. BALANCE ON TOES... KEEP
   SEAT TUCKED UNDER, BACK
   ERECT, ARMS AND THIGHS
   PARALLEL WITH FLOOR...
   HOLD ...

5. STRAIGHTEN UP SLOWLY,
   ALLOWING KNEES TO SEPARATE
   AND HEELS TO DROP ON THE
   WAY UP... COME UP WITH BACK
   ERECT...LOWER ARMS...REST.

---

## {ELBOW LOCK}

1. STRETCH ARMS FORWARD AT SHOULDER-
   LEVEL...ROLL ARMS INWARD AND
   LOCK ELBOWS...PRESS BACKS
   OF HANDS FIRMLY
   TOGETHER...FOCUS BEYOND
   HANDS... HOLD ...

2. RETURN TO A SEATED POSE..REST.

## {YOGA SEAL}

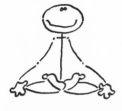 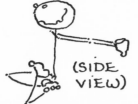 (SIDE VIEW)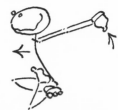

1. FROM AN EASY POSE (P. 39) OR A FULL LOTUS (P.   )... STRETCH BOTH ARMS OUT SIDEWAYS AND BEHIND BACK...

2. INTERLOCK FINGERS (WITH PALMS TOWARD BODY)... LOCK ELBOWS...KEEP SHOULDERS AS RELAXED AS POSSIBLE... <u>GENTLY</u> RAISE ARMS...

3. ROLL BODY SLOWLY FORWARD AND DOWN (LEAD WITH STERNUM)...KEEP ARMS AS HIGH AS POSSIBLE WITHOUT FORCING SHOULDERS-NECK...

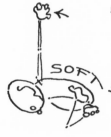

4. RELAX NECK...LAY FOREHEAD ON FLOOR (OR DROP HEAD FORWARD)... HOLD ..(CONTINUE TO RELAX BACK, LEGS AND SHOULDERS)...

5. PUSH STERNUM FORWARD AND SLOWLY STRAIGHTEN BACK...LOWER ARMS...UNLOCK FINGERS...BRING HANDS TO KNEES...REPEAT POSE, REVERSING LEGS...REST IN A SEATED POSE (P. 38).

- - - - - - - - - - - - - - - - - - - - - - - - - - - - - - - -

## {TREE 1}

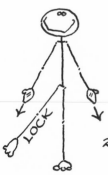

1. FROM A STANDING POSE (P. 38) SEPARATE PARALLEL FEET HIP-WIDTH APART...TURN PALMS FORWARD...STRETCH ARMS, HOLDING HANDS ABOUT 12 INCHES AWAY FROM OUTER HIPS...

2. SHIFT WEIGHT TO LEFT FOOT...LOCK BOTH KNEES...BALANCE ON LEFT FOOT AND SWING RIGHT LEG OUT SIDEWAYS...LIFT RIGHT FOOT AS HIGH AS POSSIBLE...POINT TOES...KEEP SPINE ERECT...FOCUS STRAIGHT AHEAD... HOLD ...

3. LOWER LEG AND ARMS...REPEAT POSE (OTHER SIDE)    ...REST IN A STANDING POSE.

## {WIND POSE 1}

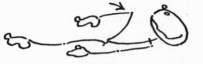 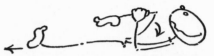

1. FROM A SUPINE POSE (P. 40) BEND RIGHT LEG... BRING RIGHT KNEE TO CHEST... INTERLOCK FINGERS OVER RIGHT SHIN CLOSE TO KNEE...

2. KEEP RIGHT HEEL BEHIND RIGHT THIGH... RELAX RIGHT HIP, LEG, FOOT... SLOWLY PULL KNEE AS CLOSE TO CHEST AS POSSIBLE... PUSH LEFT HEEL AWAY FROM BODY AND KEEP LEFT CALF ON FLOOR... TILT CHIN DOWN... FOCUS BEYOND RIGHT KNEE... HOLD ...

3. RELEASE RIGHT LEG... RETURN TO A SUPINE POSE... REPEAT POSE (OTHER SIDE), PULLING LEFT KNEE TO CHEST... REST IN A SUPINE POSE.

---

## {WIND POSE 2}

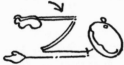 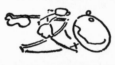 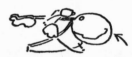

1. FROM A SUPINE POSE (P. 40) BEND LEGS AND DRAW KNEES TO CHEST... KEEP LEGS TOGETHER AND TOES EVEN...

2. FOLD FOREARMS ACROSS KNEES AND HOLD ELBOWS... RELAX LEGS AND BACK... PULL KNEES CLOSE TO CHEST...

3. SLOWLY RAISE HEAD AND TUCK NOSE BETWEEN KNEES... HOLD ...

4. LOWER HEAD TO FLOOR... UNFOLD ARMS... STRAIGHTEN LEGS... REST IN A SUPINE POSE.

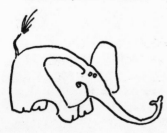

{ SPINAL TWIST 4 }

1. FROM A KNEELING POSE (P. 40 ) MOVE RIGHT FOOT FORWARD, CREATING A SQUARE-SHAPED SPACE UNDER RIGHT LEG... KEEP RIGHT HEEL IN LINE WITH RIGHT HIP...

2. SLIDE BODY FORWARD, RAISING RIGHT HEEL AND BALANCING ON TOES... KEEP LEFT KNEE AND FOOT ON FLOOR... KEEP SPINE ERECT...

3. WRAP RIGHT ARM AROUND BEHIND BACK AND HOLD UPPER LEFT ARM WITH RIGHT HAND... HOLD INNER LEFT KNEE WITH LEFT HAND... PUSH AGAINST KNEE TO TWIST CHEST AS FAR LEFT AS POSSIBLE... FOCUS ON FLOOR BEYOND LEFT FOOT... [HOLD]...

4. SWING BOTH HANDS AROUND TO RIGHT KNEE AND FACE FORWARD... PULL SLOWLY BACK INTO A KNEELING POSE... REPEAT POSE, REVERSING SIDES... REST IN A THUNDERBOLT POSE (P. 40).

-------------------------------------------------

{ CLENCH }

TILT HEAD BACKWARD AND RELAX NECK... SLOWLY OPEN MOUTH AS FAR AS POSSIBLE (WITHOUT STRAIN) AND CLOSE (AS IF CHEWING A HUGE CARAMEL).

## {EAGLE 2}

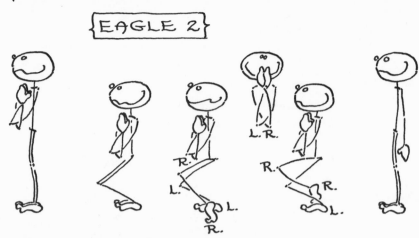

1. FROM A STANDING POSE (P.38) SEPARATE FEET 1 INCH APART...BEND LEFT ARM (PLACE HAND IN FRONT OF FACE, PALM TURNED RIGHT)...SLIP RIGHT ELBOW UNDER LEFT, AND PASS RIGHT HAND BETWEEN FACE AND LEFT HAND...LAY PALMS TOGETHER WITH THUMBS TOWARD FACE...KEEP ARMS ENTWINED AND <u>BACK ERECT</u>...

2. BEND BOTH KNEES AS DEEPLY AS POSSIBLE WITHOUT RAISING HEELS...FOCUS STRAIGHT AHEAD....

3. SHIFT BODY WEIGHT TO BENT LEFT LEG..CROSS RIGHT THIGH OVER FRONT OF LEFT THIGH.... HOOK RIGHT TOES AROUND-BEHIND ACHILLES' TENDON OF STANDING LEG...RELAX RIGHT THIGH...KEEP LEFT KNEE DEEPLY BENT AND HANDS HELD AS LOW AS POSSIBLE... HOLD ...

4. UNFOLD ARMS AND LEGS...RETURN TO A STANDING POSE...REPEAT POSE (OTHER SIDE).. REST IN A STANDING POSE.

-----------------------------------------

## {HEAD TILT 1}

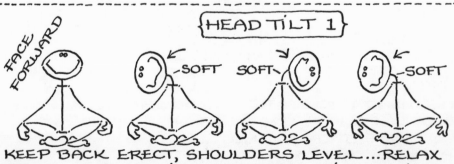

KEEP BACK ERECT, SHOULDERS LEVEL...RELAX NECK...SLOWLY TILT HEAD FROM SIDE TO SIDE... (ALLOW WEIGHT OF HEAD TO STRETCH NECK).

{ SPINAL TWIST 6 }

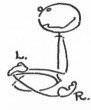 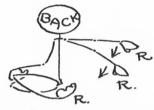 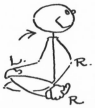

1. FROM THE HEROIC POSE (P. 41) PLACE RIGHT KNEE ON TOP OF LEFT... SIT VERY STRAIGHT AND VERY TALL DURING POSE... KEEP WEIGHT EVENLY BALANCED ON BOTH HIPS AND SHOULDERS LEVEL... HOLD RIGHT KNEE WITH LEFT HAND...

2. STRETCH RIGHT ARM AROUND BEHIND BACK AND HOLD FRONT OF RIGHT FOOT WITH RIGHT HAND (AT FIRST IT MAY NECESSARY TO LOOP A SMALL TOWEL OR SCARF OVER FOOT, IF IT IS NOT YET POSSIBLE TO REACH FOOT WITH HAND)...

3. WITH BACK ERECT, <u>BEND</u> LEFT ELBOW AND PULL GENTLY AGAINST KNEE... TURN-TWIST BODY AS FAR RIGHT AS POSSIBLE... REACH FOR CEILING WITH TOP OF HEAD... TWIST FULL LENGTH OF SPINE... FOCUS ON REAR WALL OVER RIGHT SHOULDER... [HOLD]...

4. RELEASE RIGHT FOOT AND SWING RIGHT HAND TO RIGHT KNEE... TURN FACE AND CHEST FORWARD... REPEAT POSE (OTHER SIDE) WITH LEFT KNEE ON TOP AND TWISTING LEFT... REST IN A SEATED POSE.

-------------------------------------------------

{ SHOULDER LIFT }

INHALE SLOWLY AND LIFT SHOULDERS TOWARD CEILING... EXHALE AND FLOAT SHOULDERS DOWN.

## {TORTOISE}

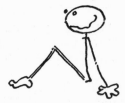 

1. FROM A SEATED POSE (P. 38)... PULL KNEES TOWARD CHEST... CREATE A RIGHT ANGLE BEHIND EACH KNEE... SEPARATE HEELS SHOULDER-WIDTH APART

2. LEAN FORWARD BETWEEN LEGS... SLIDE EACH ARM UNDER LEG (AS CLOSE TO SHOULDER AS POSSIBLE)... STRAIGHTEN ARMS... TURN PALMS DOWN... STRETCH ARMS AS FAR OUT AS POSSIBLE...

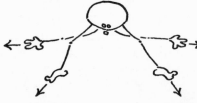 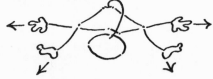

3. KEEP NECK, SHOULDERS, BACK, ABDOMEN RELAXED... SLOWLY SPREAD AND EXTEND LEGS, SLIDING ON HEELS... CREATE A RIGHT ANGLE BETWEEN LEGS...

4. STRAIGHTEN LEGS AS MUCH AS POSSIBLE... CONTINUE TO RELAX UPPER BODY... [HOLD].

5. PULL HEELS IN AGAIN TO RAISE LEGS OFF UPPER ARMS... TURN PALMS TOWARD FEET AND SLIDE ARMS OUT FROM UNDER LEGS... ROLL UP SLOWLY UNTIL BACK IS ERECT... REST IN A SEATED POSE.

- - - - - - - - - - - - - - - - - - - - - - - - - - - - - - - - - - - - -

## {DRAGONFLY}

1. EXTEND RIGHT ARM AT SHOULDER-LEVEL (PALM UP, WRIST STRAIGHT)... KEEP ELBOW IN PLACE... SWING FINGERTIPS IN A CIRCLE, CLOCKWISE AND COUNTERCLOCKWISE... BEGIN AND END CIRCLE IN LEVEL POSITION...

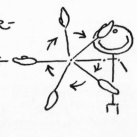

2. REPEAT CIRCLE WITH OTHER ARM.

## { SPINAL TWIST 2 }

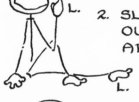

1. FROM A SEATED POSE (P. 38) BEND RIGHT LEG AND BRING KNEE TOWARD CHEST (FOOT ON FLOOR)... PLACE INNER EDGE OF RIGHT FOOT AGAINST INNER LEFT KNEE ...KEEP <u>BACK ERECT</u>, SHOULDERS LEVEL AND WEIGHT ON BOTH HIPS... <u>SIT TALL</u>...

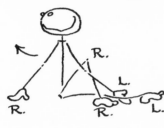

2. SLIP LEFT ELBOW OVER TO OUTSIDE OF RIGHT KNEE...PRESS ARM AGAINST LEG...

3. STRAIGHTEN LEFT ARM AND HOLD OUTER LEFT CALF WITH LEFT HAND...REACH BACK WITH RIGHT HAND AND TOUCH FINGERS ON FLOOR IN LINE WITH COCCYX... TURN AND TWIST CHEST AS FAR RIGHT AS POSSIBLE...FOCUS ON REAR WALL OVER RIGHT SHOULDER... HOLD ...

4. RELEASE LEFT CALF AND SLIP LEFT ARM OVER KNEE... STRAIGHTEN RIGHT LEG...TURN CHEST AND FACE FORWARD...BRING RIGHT HAND TO RIGHT KNEE...REPEAT POSE, REVERSING SIDES...REST IN A SEATED POSE.

- - - - - - - - - - - - - - - - - - - - - - - - - - - - - - - - - -

## { ARM TURN }

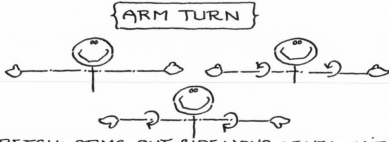

STRETCH ARMS OUT SIDEWAYS, LEVEL WITH FLOOR...KEEP SHOULDERS DOWN... SLOWLY ROTATE ARMS, TURNING PALMS FORWARD AND BACKWARD... (ARMS REMAIN FULLY STRETCHED).

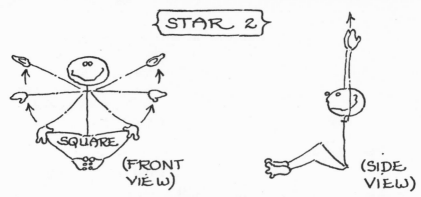

{STAR 2}

(FRONT VIEW)

(SIDE VIEW)

1. FROM A SEATED POSE (P. 38)...BEND KNEES...
BRING SOLES OF FEET TOGETHER, ALLOWING
KNEES TO DROP OUT AND DOWN...CREATE A
SQUARE-SHAPED SPACE WITHIN LEGS..
STRETCH ARMS OUT SIDEWAYS—

2. AND UP OVER HEAD TO LENGTHEN SPINE...LOOK
UP BETWEEN HANDS...ARCH SPINE BACKWARD..

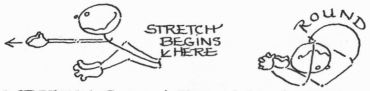

STRETCH BEGINS HERE

ROUND

3. STRETCH SLOWLY FORWARD AS FAR AS POSSIBLE
(KEEP CHIN LIFTED DURING STRETCH)...

4. INTERLOCK FINGERS AROUND TOES...PRESS
ELBOWS TO FLOOR IN FRONT OF SHINS...ROUND
BACK AS MUCH AS POSSIBLE...TOUCH TOP OF
HEAD ON FLOOR INSIDE HEELS... [HOLD]...

5. RELEASE FEET...ROLL SPINE UP SLOWLY, SLIDING
HANDS UP SHINS TO KNEES...REST IN A
SEATED POSE.

- - - - - - - - - - - - - - - - - - - - - - - - - - - - - -

{WRIST BEND}

1. STRETCH ARMS
FORWARD, LEVEL
WITH FLOOR...LOCK
ELBOWS...CREATE A RIGHT
ANGLE AT WRISTS...PUSH
PALMS FORWARD...FOCUS
BEYOND HANDS... [HOLD] WITH FINGERS UP
AND THEN WITH FINGERS POINTING DOWN...

2. RELAX ARMS...REST HANDS ON KNEES.

## { STRETCHING BREATH, LATERAL }

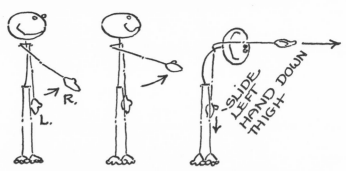

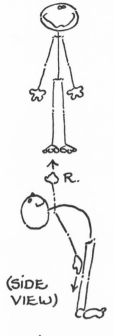

(SIDE VIEW)

1. SEPARATE PARALLEL FEET HIP-WIDTH APART IN A STANDING POSE (P. 38)...BREATHE THROUGH NOSE DURING EXERCISE...

2. RELAX ABDOMEN AND INHALE SLOWLY-DEEPLY...<u>DURING INHALATION</u>: SWING RIGHT ARM ACROSS FRONT OF BODY...REACH FOR END WALL (ARM LEVEL WITH FLOOR, IN LINE WITH LEFT ANKLE)... DURING ARM-STRETCH, TWIST HIPS LEFT TO PUSH RIGHT HIPBONE FORWARD...RELAX NECK AND WAIST...DROP HEAD BACK (EAR LEVEL WITH FLOOR)...FOCUS BEYOND RIGHT HAND...(KEEP BODY IN MOTION)...

3. <u>DURING EXHALATION</u>: SWING RIGHT ARM DOWN ACROSS FRONT OF BODY AGAIN (OVER TOES)...STRAIGHTEN AND CENTER BODY...

4. REPEAT CYCLE IMMEDIATELY BY SWINGING LEFT ARM RIGHT, ALTERNATING SIDES...BREATHE SMOOTHLY AND QUIETLY...KEEP THE MOVEMENT GRACEFUL AND FLOWING.

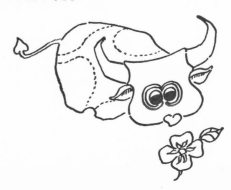

## { KNEE STRETCH }

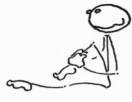

1. FROM A SEATED POSE (P. 38)... BEND RIGHT KNEE AND PULL IT TOWARD CHEST... _KEEP_ BACK ERECT AND _HIPS, LEGS, ANKLES, FEET RELAXED._...

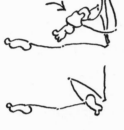

2. SLIP RIGHT ARM INSIDE RIGHT LEG... HOLD FRONT OF RIGHT _ANKLE_ WITH BOTH HANDS... PULL HEEL SLOWLY TOWARD NAVEL... LAY OUTER FOOT AND ANKLE (NOT JUST TOES) ACROSS FRONT OF UPPER LEFT THIGH (AS CLOSE TO ABDOMEN AS POSSIBLE)... ALLOW RIGHT KNEE TO DROP...

←FOCUS—

(SIDE VIEW)  (FRONT VIEW)

3. _DEEPLY RELAX_ RIGHT KNEE, ANKLE, THIGH, HIP... CUP RIGHT HAND OVER END OF RIGHT KNEE (FINGERS SPREAD)... IN ① SLOW, EVEN PUSH, PRESS RIGHT KNEE TO FLOOR (NEVER _FORCE_ KNEE!)... HOLD ...

4. LIFT RIGHT KNEE (USING HAND)... SLOWLY EXTEND RIGHT LEG... REPEAT POSE (OTHER SIDE)... REST IN A SEATED POSE.

- - - - - - - - - - - - - - - - - - - - - - - - - - - - - -

## { BRIDGE 2 }

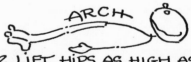

ARCH

1. FROM A SUPINE POSE (P. 40) SEPARATE FEET HIP-WIDTH APART... PLACE STRAIGHT ARMS ON FLOOR CLOSE TO BODY... KEEP ARMS AND NECK RELAXED... LOCK KNEES...

2. LIFT HIPS AS HIGH AS POSSIBLE OFF FLOOR... BALANCE ON HEELS, SHOULDERS, HEAD... FOCUS STRAIGHT UP... HOLD ...

3. SLOWLY LOWER HIPS TO FLOOR... REST IN A SUPINE POSE.

## { PILLAR }

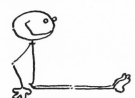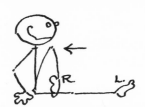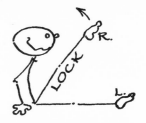

1. FROM A SEATED POSE (P. 38)... BRACE BOTH HANDS ON FLOOR BEHIND (AND CLOSE TO) HIPS...

2. BEND RIGHT KNEE...DRAW RIGHT THIGH TOWARD CHEST... KEEP LEFT LEG STRAIGHT AND ON FLOOR...

3. UNFOLD RIGHT LEG AS HIGH AS POSSIBLE...LOCK RIGHT KNEE...POINT TOES... SPINE MAY CURVE, BUT DO NOT TILT BACKWARD...FOCUS BEYOND RIGHT FOOT... HOLD

4. BRING RIGHT BENT KNEE TO CHEST...STRAIGHTEN RIGHT LEG ON FLOOR...REPEAT POSE IN REVERSE, RAISING LEFT LEG...REST IN A SEATED POSE.

---

## { HEEL TO CHEST }

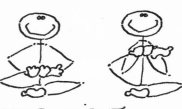

1. FROM AN EASY POSE (P. 39)... KEEP BACK ERECT AND BOTH SHOULDERS DOWN DURING POSE...SLIP HANDS UNDERNEATH OUTER RIGHT ANKLEBONE (NOT OVER FRONT OF ANKLE)... RELAX RIGHT LEG AND HIP...

2. PULL INNER RIGHT ANKLEBONE TO STERNUM... FOCUS STRAIGHT AHEAD... HOLD ...

3. LOWER RIGHT FOOT...RELEASE ANKLE... REPEAT POSE, OTHER SIDE...REST IN AN EASY POSE.

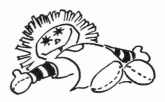

## {CAMEL 1}

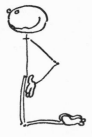
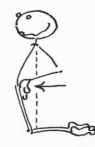

1. FROM A KNEELING POSE (P. 40)... KEEP LEGS AND FEET HIP-WIDTH APART... PLACE HANDS ON BUTTOCKS (FINGERS SPREAD)... RELAX HIPS AND SPINE...

2. KEEP HEAD <u>CENTERED</u> EXACTLY OVER SPACE BETWEEN KNEES... STEADILY PUSH ABDOMEN AS FAR FORWARD AS POSSIBLE, USING HAND PRESSURE... <u>PUSH ABDOMEN FORWARD INSTEAD OF LEANING BACKWARD</u>... FOCUS STRAIGHT AHEAD... HOLD ...

3. RETURN TO A KNEELING POSE... REST IN A THUNDERBOLT POSE.

---

## {HEAD TO KNEE 1}

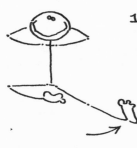

1. FROM A SEATED POSE (P. 38) BEND RIGHT LEG... PLACE RIGHT HEEL CLOSE TO GROIN... DROP RIGHT KNEE TO (OR TOWARD) FLOOR... SLIDE LEFT LEG AS FAR LEFT AS POSSIBLE... INTERLOCK FINGERS BEHIND SKULL...

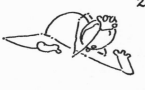

2. TURN TO FACE LEFT FOOT... STRETCH STERNUM TOWARD LEFT FOOT AND ROLL CHEST DOWN ONTO LEFT THIGH... <u>RELAX</u> NECK... PRESS BOTH ELBOWS TO (OR TOWARD) FLOOR ON EITHER SIDE OF KNEE... HOLD ...

3. RELAX ARMS... ROLL UP SLOWLY UNTIL BACK IS ERECT... FLOAT HANDS TO KNEES... RETURN TO A SEATED POSE... REPEAT POSE, (OTHER SIDE) .... REST IN A SEATED POSE.

## { HALF TORTOISE }

1. FROM A THUNDERBOLT POSE (P. 40) REACH OUT SIDEWAYS AND UP OVER HEAD... JOIN PALMS, CROSS THUMBS... STRETCH UP TO <u>LOCK</u> <u>ELBOWS</u> IN AGAINST HEAD... <u>HIPS</u> <u>MUST</u> <u>REMAIN</u> <u>ON</u> <u>HEELS</u> DURING ENTIRE POSE...

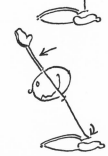

2. REACH SLOWLY FORWARD AND DOWN, WITHOUT LIFTING HIPS OFF HEELS... (STRETCH SHOULD TRAVEL FROM COCCYX THROUGH ———→ FINGERTIPS)...

3. TOUCH LITTLE FINGERS ON FLOOR... KEEPING ELBOWS TIGHTLY LOCKED, AND HEAD BETWEEN ARMS— SLiiiiiiDE LITTLE FINGERS AS FAR FORWARD AS POSSIBLE (DO NOT ALLOW WRISTS TO TOUCH FLOOR)...

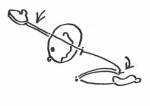

4. AT FURTHEST POINT OF STRETCH, LEAVE <u>ARMS</u> <u>LOCKED</u> AND REST FOREHEAD ON FLOOR... [ HOLD ]...

5. PLACE HEAD BETWEEN ARMS AGAIN... <u>WITHOUT</u> <u>LIFTING</u> <u>HIPS</u> <u>OFF</u> <u>HEELS</u>, SIT UP (REACHING FOR CEILING)... SEPARATE HANDS, BRING THEM DOWN SIDEWAYS TO KNEES... REST IN A THUNDERBOLT POSE.

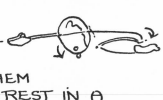

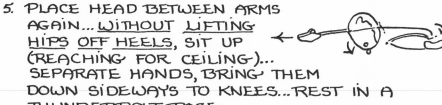

## { HEAD TO KNEE 4 }

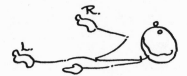 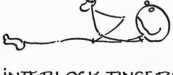

1 FROM A SUPINE POSE (P. 40)..BEND RIGHT LEG... DRAW KNEE TO CHEST...

2. INTERLOCK FINGERS BEHIND TOES (AVOID ARCH)... KEEP LEFT LEG ON FLOOR...

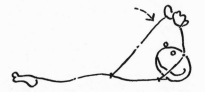 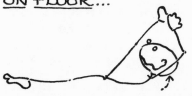

3 SLOWLY UNFOLD RIGHT LEG, STRAIGHT UP...LOCK RIGHT KNEE...BEND BOTH ELBOWS TO PULL RIGHT FOOT BACK OVER HEAD...

4. CONTINUE TO BEND ELBOWS...RAISE HEAD... BRING FACE TO RIGHT LEG...FOCUS BEYOND INNER RIGHT KNEE... HOLD ...

5. LOWER HEAD TO FLOOR...BEND KNEE...RELEASE FOOT...RETURN RIGHT LEG TO FLOOR...REPEAT POSE (OTHER SIDE)..REST IN A SUPINE POSE.

---

## { PELVIC TILT }

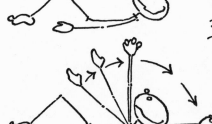

1. FROM A SUPINE POSE (P. 40) KEEP LEGS TOGETHER AND BEND KNEES INTO A RIGHT ANGLE..

2. REACH UP OVER FACE... INTERLOCK FINGERS... LOCK ELBOWS...BRING HANDS TO FLOOR OVER HEAD... KEEP NECK AND SHOULDERS RELAXED...

3. TUCK SEAT UNDER..PULL NAVEL TOWARD CHEST... KEEP FULL SPINE ON FLOOR...FOCUS.. HOLD ...

4. BRING HANDS OVER FACE, UNLACE FINGERS, LOWER ARMS BY SIDES...STRAIGHTEN LEGS... REST.

## { LOTUS BLOSSOMING }

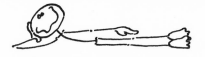 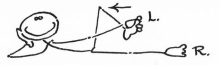

1. FROM A SIDE-LYING POSE, LYING ON RIGHT SIDE (P. 39)...

2. BEND LEFT LEG...BRING LEFT KNEE TOWARD HEAD... SLIP FIRST 2 FINGERS OF LEFT HAND AROUND LEFT BIG TOE...(PALM SHOULD BE TURNED FORWARD)... KEEP RIGHT LEG ON FLOOR (KNEE LOCKED, TOES POINTED)...

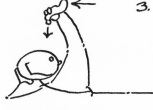

3. SLOWLY UNFOLD LEFT LEG STRAIGHT UP...LOCK LEFT KNEE AND PULL TOES TOWARD HEAD...BEND LEFT ELBOW TO DRAW LEFT FOOT BACK OVER HEAD AS FAR AS POSSIBLE... FOCUS BEYOND RIGHT FOOT... HOLD ...

4. BEND LEFT KNEE, RELEASE FOOT...EXTEND LEFT LEG...ROLL OVER ON LEFT SIDE AND REPEAT POSE, OTHER SIDE....REST IN A SUPINE POSE (P. 40).

- - - - - - - - - - - - - - - - - - - - - - - - - - - - - - -

## { ATLAS BEND }

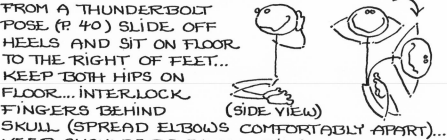

1. FROM A THUNDERBOLT POSE (P. 40) SLIDE OFF HEELS AND SIT ON FLOOR TO THE RIGHT OF FEET... KEEP BOTH HIPS ON FLOOR...INTERLOCK FINGERS BEHIND (SIDE VIEW) SKULL (SPREAD ELBOWS COMFORTABLY APART)...

2. KEEP SHOULDERS EQUAL DISTANCE FROM FRONT WALL...TILT BODY OVER FEET..RELAX RIGHT SIDE AND ALLOW GRAVITY TO LOWER ELBOW TO FLOOR...FOCUS STRAIGHT AHEAD... HOLD ...

3 ROLL UP SLOWLY...BRING HANDS TO KNEES AND SIT ON OTHER SIDE OF HEELS... REPEAT POSE (OTHER SIDE)...REST IN AN EASY POSE (P. 39).

## {SEATED FROG}

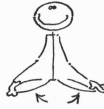 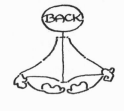 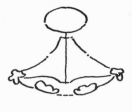

1. FROM A THUNDERBOLT POSE (P.40) SPREAD KNEES AS FAR APART AS POSSIBLE...

2. SEPARATE TIPS OF BIG TOES JUST ENOUGH TO ALLOW HIPS TO REST FIRMLY ON FLOOR INSIDE OF FEET... (INNER CURVE OF FOOT SHOULD LIE CLOSE TO OUTER CURVE OF HIP)...RELAX FEET, ANKLES, KNEES AND ALLOW GRAVITY TO LOWER HIPS TO FLOOR (DO NOT FORCE KNEES OR BOUNCE!!!)...

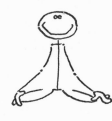

3. SIT STRAIGHT AND TALL...REST HANDS ON KNEES...FOCUS STRAIGHT AHEAD... HOLD ...

4. BRACE HANDS ON FLOOR NEAR HIPS...CENTER KNEES AGAIN (1 AT A TIME)...REST IN A THUNDERBOLT POSE.

---------------------------------------------------

## {SPINAL TWIST 1}

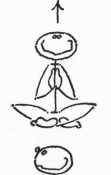

1. FROM AN EASY POSE (P.39) JOIN PALMS IN FRONT OF CHEST AND REST ARMS AGAINST SIDES...SIT TALL-TALL-TALL-TALL...RELAX SHOULDERS...SIT EVENLY ON BOTH HIPS...KEEP BACK ERECT, THUMBS ON STERNUM, CHIN EXACTLY OVER FINGERTIPS DURING COMPLETE POSE...

2. ROTATE AND TWIST SPINE, TURNING AS FAR RIGHT AS POSSIBLE...FOCUS IN LINE WITH STERNUM... HOLD ...

3. TURN FACE AND CHEST FORWARD AGAIN... COMPLETE POSE BY TWISTING LEFT...REST IN AN EASY POSE.

## { BOAT WITH OARS }

STRAIGHT

1. FROM A SEATED POSE (P.38)... BEND LEGS AND KEEP FEET TOGETHER... TOUCH FINGERS LIGHTLY TO FLOOR OPPOSITE HIPS... BALANCE BETWEEN COCCYX AND SACRUM... KEEP SPINE STRAIGHT AND STERNUM GENTLY LIFTED...
2. UNFOLD LEGS AT A 60° ANGLE TO FLOOR... LOCK KNEES AND POINT TOES... BALANCE...
3. STRETCH ARMS FORWARD, LEVEL WITH FLOOR, PALMS DOWN... (FEET SHOULD BE HIGHER THAN HEAD)... FOCUS BEYOND FEET... |HOLD|...
4. BEND KNEES... LOWER FEET TO FLOOR... REST IN A SEATED POSE.

------------------------------------------------

## { COBRA 1 }

SOFT TIGHT

(KEEP LEGS TOGETHER, FEET ON FLOOR.)

1. FROM A PRONE POSE (P.38)... FOLD ARMS ON FLOOR IN FRONT OF CHEST... HOLD OPPOSITE ELBOWS... REST FOREHEAD ON ARMS... KEEP LEG ←—FOCUS— MUSCLES TIGHT...
2. PRESS ELBOWS AGAINST FLOOR AND LIFT CHEST AS HIGH AS POSSIBLE... KEEP SHOULDERS DOWN AND RELAXED, STERNUM LIFTED, NECK ↓ LONG, FACE SERENE... FOCUS STRAIGHT AHEAD.. |HOLD|... (IT IS VERY IMPORTANT TO KEEP SHOULDER MUSCLES PULLED AWAY FROM NECK)..
3. SLOWLY LOWER CHEST AND LAY HEAD ON FOLDED ARMS... REST IN A PRONE POSE.

{ HALF LOCUST 1 }

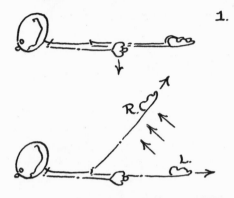

1. FROM A PRONE POSE (P. 38 ) BRING LEGS TOGETHER...POINT TOES ...LOCK KNEES...LOCK ELBOWS...PRESS FISTS AGAINST FLOOR, CLOSE TO BODY (THUMB AND INDEX FINGER DOWN)... STRETCH FACE FORWARD...REST POINT OF CHIN ON FLOOR...

2. KEEP BOTH LEGS STRETCHED – STRAIGHT... SLOWLY RAISE STRAIGHT RIGHT LEG AS HIGH AS POSSIBLE (KEEP FULL LENGTH OF LEFT LEG ON FLOOR)... DO NOT SWING RIGHT LEG OVER LEFT AND KEEP KNEECAP TURNED DOWN...FOCUS ON FLOOR... HOLD ...

3. SLOWLY LOWER RIGHT LEG TO FLOOR ... REPEAT POSE, RAISING LEFT LEG...REST IN A PRONE POSE.

-----------------------------------------

{ HALF LOCUST 2 }

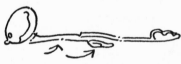 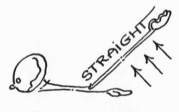

1. FROM A PRONE POSE (P. 38) KEEP LEGS TOGETHER, KNEES LOCKED, TOES POINTED... STRETCH FACE FORWARD...REST POINT OF CHIN (OR MOUTH) ON FLOOR... LOCK ELBOWS AND TUCK STRAIGHT ARMS UNDER BODY (PALMS DOWN, LITTLE FINGERS TOGETHER)...

2. SHIFT BALANCE FORWARD TO ARMS-CHEST... PRESS HANDS AGAINST FLOOR...IN A QUICK (BUT SMOOTH) MOVEMENT, LIFT BOTH LEGS AS HIGH AS POSSIBLE... HOLD ...

3. SLOWLY LOWER LEGS TO FLOOR... FREE ARMS...REST IN A PRONE POSE.

(OMIT POSE DURING ANY STAGE OF PREGNANCY.....)

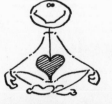

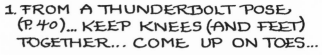

## {RABBIT}

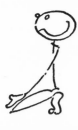

1. FROM A THUNDERBOLT POSE (P. 40)... KEEP KNEES (AND FEET) TOGETHER... COME UP ON TOES...

2. FIRMLY GRASP ARCH OF EACH FOOT (1 AT A TIME)... TUCK CHIN ON CHEST... ROUND BACK AS MUCH AS POSSIBLE FROM COCCYX TO HEAD... PULL ABDOMINAL WALL IN TOWARD SPINE... ROLL SLOWLY FORWARD...

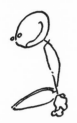

3. BRING FOREHEAD TO KNEES (ARMS WILL STRETCH OUT STRAIGHT AND HIPS WILL LIFT OFF HEELS)... <u>DO NOT ALLOW HEAD TO TOUCH FLOOR</u>... [HOLD]...

ROUND

4. SIT BACK ON HEELS AND ROLL UP SLOWLY (1 VERTEBRA AT A TIME)... RELEASE FEET... REST IN A THUNDERBOLT POSE.

---

## {BRIDGE 1}

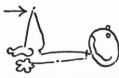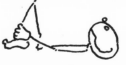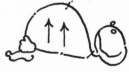

1. BEND KNEES AND BRING FEET CLOSE TO HIPS... PLACE EACH OUTER ANKLEBONE IN LINE WITH OUTER CURVE OF HIP... KEEP HEELS ON FLOOR AND FEET PARALLEL...

2. HOLD FRONTS OF ANKLES (OR LEAVE ARMS ON FLOOR CLOSE TO BODY, PALMS DOWN)...

3. SLOWLY-SMOOTHLY ARCH SPINE... RAISE ABDOMEN AS HIGH AS POSSIBLE... BALANCE ON FEET, SHOULDERS, AND HEAD (<u>KEEP NECK AND SHOULDERS</u> RELAXED).. FOCUS ON CEILING... [HOLD]...

4. SLOWLY FLOAT HIPS DOWN TO FLOOR... RELEASE ANKLES AND STRAIGHTEN LEGS... REST IN A SUPINE POSE.

## {WALL-REST}

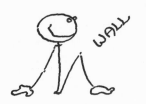

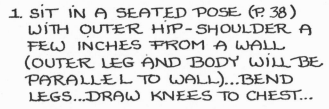

1. SIT IN A SEATED POSE (P. 38) WITH OUTER HIP-SHOULDER A FEW INCHES FROM A WALL (OUTER LEG AND BODY WILL BE PARALLEL TO WALL)...BEND LEGS...DRAW KNEES TO CHEST...

2. USING HANDS AND ELBOWS FOR BALANCE, PIVOT ON LOWER SPINE TO FACE WALL...UNFOLD LEGS...REST HEELS AGAINST WALL (HIP-WIDTH APART)...HIPS SHOULD BE FAR ENOUGH FROM WALL TO ALLOW LEGS TO COMPLETELY RELAX IN PLACE... SPREAD ARMS OUT SIDEWAYS (PALMS UP)...

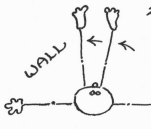

3. CLOSE EYES AND RELAX NECK, SPINE, SHOULDERS, LEGS... BREATHE DEEPLY, QUIETLY... HOLD ...

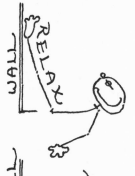

4. SLOWLY DRAW KNEES TO CHEST AND FOLD LEFT ARM-HAND OVER SHINS...ROLL OVER TOWARD EXTENDED RIGHT ARM AND REST IN PLACE, AT LEAST 30 SECONDS...REST IN A SEATED POSE.

- - - - - - - - - - - - - - - - - - - - - - - - - - - - - -

## {FOLDED LEAF}

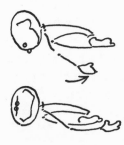

1. FROM A THUNDERBOLT POSE (P. 40) LAY CHEST ON THIGHS...REST HANDS (PALMS UP) ON FLOOR NEAR FEET,.. KEEP HIPS ON HEELS...

2. TURN SIDE OF HEAD TO REST ON FLOOR IN FRONT OF KNEES... CLOSE EYES...RELAX ENTIRE BODY...HOLD ...

3. ROLL UP (1 VERTEBRA AT A TIME) UNTIL BACK IS ERECT... RAISE FACE AGAIN...RETURN HANDS TO KNEES...REST IN A THUNDERBOLT POSE.

## SPINAL COLUMN POSE 2

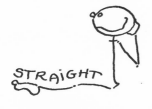

STRAIGHT

(TREMBLING IS NATURAL AT FIRST)

1. FROM A SEATED POSE (P. 38) KEEP KNEES LOCKED, TOES POINTED, <u>FEET</u> <u>ON</u> <u>FLOOR</u>, LEGS TOGETHER, SPINE AND NECK STRAIGHT... INTERLOCK FINGERS BEHIND SKULL...

2. SPREAD ELBOWS A COMFORTABLE DISTANCE APART... TILT BODY BACKWARD TO A 45° ANGLE... FOCUS AND HOLD ...

3. SLOWLY SIT UP STRAIGHT...BRING HANDS TO KNEES...REST IN A SEATED POSE.

------------------------------------------------

## CRADLE

1. FROM AN EASY POSE (P. 39) HOLD FRONT OF RIGHT ANKLE WITH RIGHT HAND... LAY OUTER EDGE OF FOOT IN INNER BEND OF LEFT ELBOW... ALLOW TOES AND BALL OF FOOT TO EXTEND BEYOND ELBOW...RELAX RIGHT LEG AND KEEP <u>BACK</u> <u>ERECT</u>...

2. WRAP RIGHT ARM AROUND RIGHT KNEE... ALLOW KNEE TO EXTEND BEYOND INNER ELBOW...INTERLOCK FINGERS OUTSIDE LOWER RIGHT LEG...PULL IN LOWER LEG TO TOUCH CHEST...FOCUS STRAIGHT AHEAD. HOLD

3. UNLOCK FINGERS... AGAIN HOLD RIGHT ANKLE WITH RIGHT HAND...FREE LEFT ARM...LOWER LEG...REPEAT POSE (OTHER SIDE), HOLDING LEFT LEG...REST IN AN EASY POSE.

{ BACK STRETCH 1 }

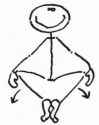

(FRONT VIEW)

1. FROM A SEATED POSE (P. 38)... BEND KNEES... TURN SOLES OF FEET TOGETHER... RELAX LEGS, ALLOWING KNEES TO DROP OUTWARD...

(SIDE VIEW)

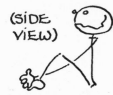

2. CREATE A SQUARE-SHAPED SPACE WITHIN BENT LEGS... REACH BETWEEN KNEES TO FIRMLY HOLD RIGHT TOES WITH RIGHT HAND, LEFT TOES WITH LEFT HAND...

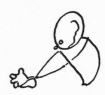

3. DROP BODY FORWARD AND DOWN BETWEEN LEGS, RELAXING FACE, NECK, SHOULDERS AND SPINE AS MUCH AS POSSIBLE...

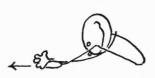

4. SLIDE OUTER EDGES OF FEET FORWARD ALONG THE FLOOR (AWAY FROM BODY)... KEEP UPPER BODY COMPLETELY RELAXED...

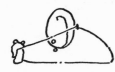

5. STRAIGHTEN LEGS... SEPARATE SOLES OF FEET AND GRADUALLY TURN THEM FORWARD... (ARMS WILL BE STRETCHED STRAIGHT)..

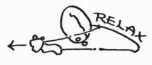

6. SLOWLY POINT TOES... ALLOW FORWARD THRUST OF TOES TO STRETCH SHOULDERS AND BACK... FOCUS ON FLOOR... HOLD ...

7. ROLL UP SLOWLY, 1 VERTEBRA AT A TIME... SLIDE HANDS UP SHINS TO KNEES... REST IN A SEATED POSE.

## { SPINAL COLUMN POSE 1 }

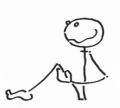 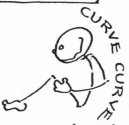 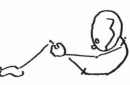

CURVE CURVE

1. FROM A SEATED POSE (P.38)... KEEP FEET ON FLOOR, LEGS TOGETHER... BEND KNEES TO CREATE A RIGHT ANGLE BEHIND EACH KNEE... TOUCH <u>VERY LIGHTLY</u> THE BACK OF EACH THIGH, CLOSE TO KNEE...

2. TUCK CHIN ON CHEST AND <u>CURVE ENTIRE SPINE</u> AS MUCH AS POSSIBLE... ROLL SLOWLY BACKWARD TO LAY <u>SACRUM</u> ON FLOOR... LET ABDOMINAL MUSCLES HOLD BODY IN PLACE... FOCUS ON ABDOMEN... [HOLD]...

3. SIT UP SLOWLY... REST IN A SEATED POSE.

---

## { BOW 1 }

1. FROM A PRONE POSE (P. 38)... BEND LEGS AND BRING HEELS TO HIPS (KNEES HIP-WIDTH APART)...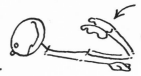

2. HOLD FRONT OF EACH ANKLE (OR FOOT)... HOLD EACH FOOT IN EXACTLY THE SAME PLACE... KEEP THUMB AND FINGERS TOGETHER... RELAX NECK, SHOULDERS, LUMBAR...

3. SMOOTHLY KICK <u>STRAIGHT UP</u> AS HIGH AS POSSIBLE... <u>KEEP UPPER BODY PASSIVE</u>... FOCUS STRAIGHT AHEAD... KEEP NECK RELAXED... [HOLD]...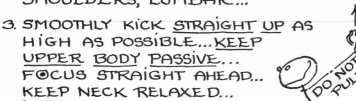

DO NOT PULL

4. RELAX KICK, LOWER KNEES, RELEASE FEET... REST IN A PRONE POSE.

(OMIT POSE DURING ANY STAGE OF PREGNANCY.....)

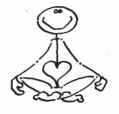

{ COBRA 2 }

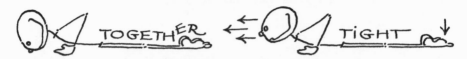

1. FROM A PRONE POSE (P.38) PLACE HANDS
   (PALMS DOWN) UNDERNEATH SHOULDERS...
   POINT FINGERS FORWARD (WITH EACH LITTLE
   FINGER IN LINE WITH OUTER SHOULDER
   AND FINGERTIPS IN LINE WITH TOP OF
   SHOULDER)...LOCK KNEES...POINT TOES...<u>KEEP
   FEET ON FLOOR, LEGS TOGETHER, BUTTOCKS
   MUSCLES TIGHT</u>...REST FOREHEAD ON FLOOR...

2. SLIDE CHEST AND FACE FORWARD ALONG
   FLOOR...RELAX AND LOWER SHOULDERS...

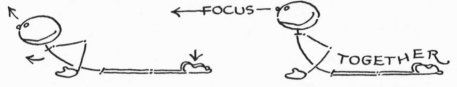

3. PUSH STERNUM GENTLY FORWARD...RAISE
   CHEST ENOUGH TO LIFT NAVEL OFF FLOOR.
   AND TO CREATE A <u>RIGHT ANGLE BEND</u> WITH
   EACH ELBOW...<u>PRESS ARMS AGAINST BODY</u>...

4. FOCUS STRAIGHT AHEAD..."FLOAT" SKULL
   ABOVE NECK...PULL SHOULDERS DOWN AWAY
   FROM HEAD (THERE SHOULD BE NO SKIN-
   CREASE BETWEEN BASE OF NECK AND
   SHOULDER)...TRY TO KEEP BODY IN PLACE
   WITH BACK MUSCLES RATHER THAN ARM
   STRENGTH... [HOLD] ...

5. GENTLY PULL FACE
   AND STERNUM
   FORWARD... SLOWLY
   ROLL FRONT OF
   BODY DOWN ONTO FLOOR...
   (KEEP NECK LONG AND SHOULDERS DOWN)..
   REST IN A PRONE POSE.

## {PELVIC STRETCH}

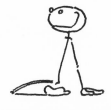

1. FROM A THUNDERBOLT POSE (P40) TILT SLIGHTLY BACKWARD AND PUT PALMS ON FLOOR (ABOUT 4 INCHES BEYOND TOES)...POINT FINGERS STRAIGHT BACK (THUMBS IN LINE WITH OUTER HIPS)... KEEP KNEES TOGETHER, ARMS STRAIGHT, HANDS IN PLACE...

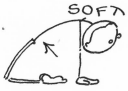

SOFT

2. SLOWLY RAISE HIPS OFF HEELS AND LIFT ABDOMEN AS FAR FORWARD AND UP AS POSSIBLE...RELAX NECK TO SLOWLY DROP HEAD BACKWARD. FOCUS ON REAR WALL... PRESS SHOULDERS TOWARD KNEES AND CONTINUE TO RELAX NECK... HOLD ...

3. "FLOAT" HIPS DOWN TO HEELS, CAREFULLY RAISING HEAD... SWING HANDS AROUND TO REST ON KNEES...REST IN A THUNDERBOLT POSE.

---

## {BALANCED BACK STRETCH}

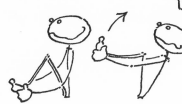

1. FROM A SEATED POSE (P. 38) DRAW BENT KNEES TOWARD CHEST (FEET ON FLOOR, LEGS TOGETHER)... KEEP BACK STRAIGHT AND STERNUM LIFTED...

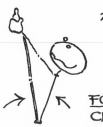

2. TIGHTLY GRASP HEELS (OR OUTER CALVES)...BALANCE ON COCCYX... LIFT FEET OFF FLOOR...UNFOLD LEGS STRAIGHT UP...LOCK KNEES... PRESS ABDOMINAL WALL GENTLY FORWARD...BRING BODY AND LEGS AS CLOSE TOGETHER AS POSSIBLE... FOCUS BEYOND TOES... HOLD ...

3. SLOWLY BEND LEGS, BRING KNEES TO CHEST, LOWER FEET TO FLOOR...RELEASE HEELS... EXTEND LEGS...REST IN A SEATED POSE.

## { STANDING REST }

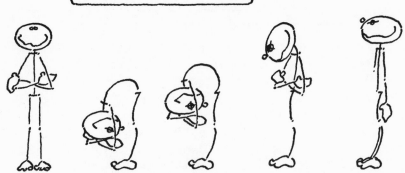

1. FROM A STANDING POSE (P. 38)... CROSS FOREARMS IN FRONT OF BODY... TUCK EACH HAND IN BEND OF OPPOSITE ELBOW... GENTLY LOCK KNEES...

2. ROLL SLOWLY FORWARD AND DOWN, RELAXING DEEPLY ARMS, SHOULDERS, NECK, SPINE, ABDOMINAL WALL... CLOSE EYES... (BOTH ELBOWS DROP STRAIGHT DOWN)... HOLD ...

3. ROLL UP SLOWLY (1 VERTEBRA AT A TIME)... RETURN TO A STANDING POSE, CONTINUING TO REST ARMS AGAINST BODY AND CHIN ON CHEST... REMAIN IN THIS POSITION AT LEAST 30 SECONDS LONGER... OPEN EYES... LOWER ARMS.

------

## { INCLINED PLANE }

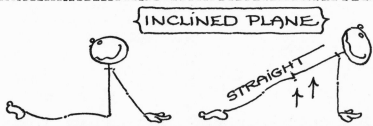

STRAIGHT

1. FROM A SEATED POSE (P. 38)... PLACE PALMS ON FLOOR BEHIND HIPS (FINGERS POINTING BACK- WARD, THUMBS IN LINE WITH OUTER HIPS)... LOCK ELBOWS AND KNEES... POINT TOES...

2. LIFT ABDOMEN TOWARD CEILING TO BRING LEGS - BODY - NECK ALL IN 1 STRAIGHT LINE... ARMS SHOULD BE PERPENDICULAR TO FLOOR.. FOCUS ON CEILING... HOLD ...

3. FLOAT HIPS TO FLOOR... RETURN HANDS TO KNEES... REST IN A SEATED POSE.

## {WINGED BREATH}

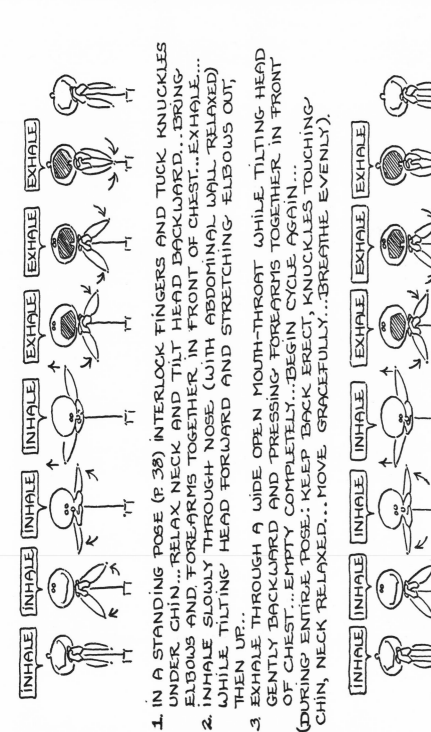

1. IN A STANDING POSE (P. 38) INTERLOCK FINGERS AND TUCK KNUCKLES UNDER CHIN...RELAX NECK AND TILT HEAD BACKWARD...BRING ELBOWS AND FOREARMS TOGETHER IN FRONT OF CHEST...EXHALE...

2. INHALE SLOWLY THROUGH NOSE (WITH ABDOMINAL WALL RELAXED) WHILE TILTING HEAD FORWARD AND STRETCHING ELBOWS OUT, THEN UP...

3. EXHALE THROUGH A WIDE OPEN MOUTH-THROAT WHILE TILTING HEAD GENTLY BACKWARD AND PRESSING FOREARMS TOGETHER IN FRONT OF CHEST...EMPTY COMPLETELY...BEGIN CYCLE AGAIN...

(DURING ENTIRE POSE: KEEP BACK ERECT, KNUCKLES TOUCHING CHIN, NECK RELAXED...MOVE GRACEFULLY...BREATHE EVENLY).

## {INTENSE SIDE STRETCH}

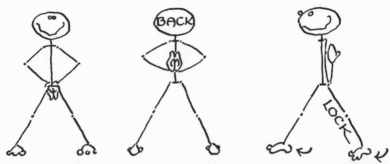

1. SEPARATE PARALLEL FEET 3 FEET APART IN A SPREAD FOOT POSE (P. 39)... BRING ARMS BEHIND BACK...JOIN PALMS BEHIND SACRUM...

2. TURN FINGERTIPS FIRST IN TOWARD SPINE, THEN UP TOWARD HEAD... SLIDE LITTLE FINGERS UP SPINE AS FAR AS POSSIBLE... RELAX SHOULDERS... (AT FIRST IT MAY BE DIFFICULT TO JOIN PALMS...IF SO, JUST HOLD OPPOSITE ELBOWS)...

3. TURN RIGHT INTO AN ANGLED FOOT POSE (P. 41) BRINGING STERNUM IN LINE WITH RIGHT SHIN... LOCK KNEES...KEEP THIGH MUSCLES <u>TIGHT</u> DURING ENTIRE POSE...

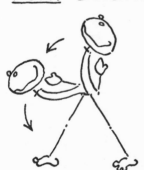

4. TILT HEAD BACKWARD...GENTLY STRETCH CHIN AND STERNUM OUT OVER RIGHT LEG (AS IF TO TOUCH CHIN ON END WALL)... CONTINUE THE STRETCH, BRINGING THE CHIN TOWARD RIGHT SHIN... KEEP PALMS TOGETHER...

5. LENGTHEN SPINE AS MUCH AS POSSIBLE... RELAX NECK AND LET HEAD HANG...KEEP SHOULDERS LEVEL, KNEES LOCKED, STERNUM OVER SHIN...FOCUS BEYOND KNEE... HOLD ...

6. GRACEFULLY STRETCH CHIN TOWARD END WALL AND STRAIGHTEN BACK...TURN BODY AND TOES FORWARD... RELAX SHOULDERS... REPEAT POSE, TURNING LEFT... SLOWLY SLIDE HANDS DOWN SPINE AND REST IN A STANDING POSE...

## { MOON POSE }

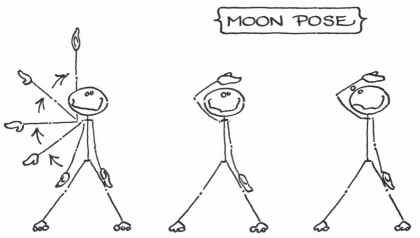

1. FROM A SPREAD FOOT POSE (P. 39) SEPARATE FEET 3 FEET APART... KEEP KNEES LOCKED AND FEET PARALLEL... STRETCH RIGHT ARM OUT SIDEWAYS AND UP OVER HEAD...

2. BEND RIGHT ELBOW AND "FLOAT" PALM OVER TOP OF HEAD...

3. TURN FACE TOWARD INNER ELBOW... KEEP NECK AND SHOULDERS AS RELAXED AS POSSIBLE...

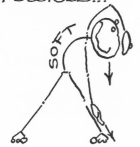

4. SLIDE LEFT PALM DOWN OUTSIDE LEFT LEG AS FAR AS POSSIBLE... (KEEP BACK AND HIPS TOUCHING IMAGINARY WALL)... KEEP PALM OVER TOP OF HEAD... FOCUS ON CEILING BEYOND INNER ELBOW... ELBOW AND NOSE SHOULD POINT STRAIGHT UP... HOLD ...

5. STRAIGHTEN UP SLOWLY... TOUCH CEILING WITH RIGHT HAND... BRING RIGHT HAND DOWN TO RIGHT LEG... TURN FACE FORWARD... REPEAT POSE, (OTHER SIDE)., SLIDING RIGHT HAND DOWN RIGHT LEG... REST IN A STANDING POSE (P. 38).

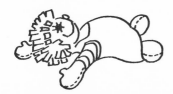

{EAGLE 1}

1 FROM A STANDING POSE
(P. 38) SEPARATE FEET 1
INCH... JOIN PALMS IN FRONT
OF CHEST... REST ELBOWS
AGAINST SIDES... KEEP BACK
ERECT, SHOULDERS LEVEL
(AND EXACTLY SAME
DISTANCE FROM FRONT WALL)
BEND BOTH KNEES AS DEEPLY
AS POSSIBLE, KEEPING HEELS ON
FLOOR... FOCUS STRAIGHT AHEAD....

2 SHIFT BODY WEIGHT TO BENT LEFT LEG...
CROSS RIGHT THIGH OVER FRONT OF LEFT
THIGH AND TOUCH RIGHT BIG TOE ON FLOOR
OUTSIDE LEFT FOOT... DO NOT TWIST SPINE...
HOLD ...

3 UNCROSS AND STRAIGHTEN LEGS... LOWER
ARMS... REPEAT POSE (OTHER SIDE)... REST IN A
STANDING POSE.

--------------------------------------------------

{SERPENT}

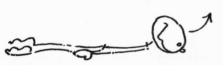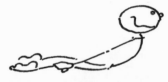

1. FROM A PRONE POSE (P. 38) SEPARATE FEET
HIP-WIDTH APART... POINT TOES... LAY HANDS
(PALMS DOWN) ON BACKS OF THIGHS OR HIPS...
KEEP FEET ON FLOOR AND ARMS STRAIGHT...

2. SLOWLY SLIDE FACE AND CHEST FORWARD ALONG
FLOOR AND RAISE CHEST AS HIGH AS
POSSIBLE (ALL IN 1 GRACEFUL MOVEMENT)...
SLIDE HANDS DOWN LEGS TOWARD HEELS...
KEEP SHOULDERS RELAXED AND DOWN...
HEAD SHOULD "FLOAT" ABOVE A GENTLY
STRETCHED NECK... FOCUS STRAIGHT AHEAD...
HOLD ...

3. SLOWLY ROLL BODY FORWARD AND DOWN
(1 VERTEBRA AT A TIME)... REST IN A PRONE
POSE.

## {THE SUN, RISING}

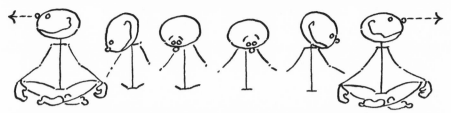

1. FROM AN EASY POSE (P. 39)...KEEP SHOULDERS LEVEL, BACK ERECT, STERNUM SLIGHTLY LIFTED, NECK RELAXED DURING ENTIRE POSE... TURN HEAD RIGHT...FOCUS BEYOND RIGHT SHOULDER... HOLD ...LOWER POINT OF CHIN TO FAR END OF RIGHT CLAVICLE... SLOOOWLY SLIDE CHIN LEFT ACROSS CHEST TO FAR END OF LEFT CLAVICLE ...RAISE FACE...FOCUS BEYOND LEFT SHOULDER.. HOLD

2. LOWER CHIN TO END OF LEFT CLAVICLE... SLIDE CHIN TO CENTER THROAT...RAISE FACE...REST.

---

## {SEPARATE LEG STRETCH}

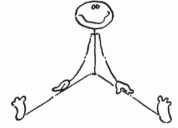 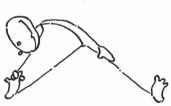

1. FROM A SEATED POSE (P. 38)... SPREAD LEGS AS FAR APART AS POSSIBLE...KEEP KNEES LOCKED...

2. SLIP FIRST 2 FINGERS OF EACH HAND BETWEEN BIG TOE AND SECOND TOE (PALMS TURNED IN)...

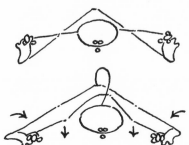

3. COMPLETELY RELAX NECK, FACE, SPINE, ABDOMINAL WALL... (LEGS REMAIN STRAIGHT)...

4. SLOWLY PULL BIG TOES IN AND DOWN TO TOUCH FLOOR.. PRESS ELBOWS TO FLOOR NEAR INNER KNEES. HOLD . (ALLOW HEAD TO HANG)... FOCUS ON FLOOR...

5. RELEASE TOES...ROLL SPINE UP SLOWLY...SLIDE HANDS TO KNEES...REST IN A SEATED POSE.

## { ARM MOTION }

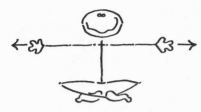 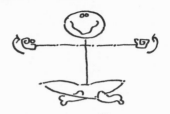

1. FROM AN EASY POSE (P. 39) EXTEND ARMS OUT SIDEWAYS AT SHOULDER LEVEL, PALMS UP...

2. MAKE A TIGHT FIST WITH EACH HAND... KEEP UPPER ARMS LEVEL WITH FLOOR...

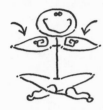

3. BEND ELBOWS... BRING FISTS IN TO TOUCH SHOULDERS... KEEP FISTS TIGHT, BACK STRAIGHT... CONTRACT EVERY ARM MUSCLE... FOCUS STRAIGHT AHEAD... [HOLD] ...

4. EXTEND ARMS AGAIN... RELAX AND OPEN HANDS... REST HANDS ON KNEES.

---

## { HALF MOON 2 }

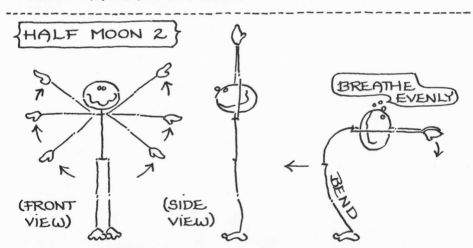

(FRONT VIEW)  (SIDE VIEW)  BREATHE EVENLY  BEND

1. FROM A STANDING POSE (P. 38)... SEPARATE FEET HIP-DISTANCE APART... STRETCH ARMS OUT AND UP... JOIN PALMS OVER HEAD... LOCK ELBOWS...

2. PUSH HIPS AS FAR FORWARD AS POSSIBLE... UNLOCK KNEES... LAY ARMS/HEAD GENTLY BACK (RELAX NECK)... FOCUS ON CEILING... [HOLD]...

3. REACH UP TO CEILING AGAIN TO STRAIGHTEN BACK AND RAISE FACE... LOWER ARMS SIDEWAYS AND DOWN... REST IN A STANDING POSE.

## {ANKLE BALANCE 1}

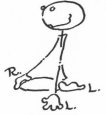

1. FROM A THUNDERBOLT POSE (P. 40)... TOUCH LEFT HAND LIGHTLY ON FLOOR OPPOSITE LEFT HIP... KEEP SPINE ERECT, SHOULDERS LEVEL, FEET AND ANKLES COMPLETELY RELAXED... HOLD FRONT OF RIGHT KNEE WITH RIGHT HAND... FOCUS STRAIGHT AHEAD.

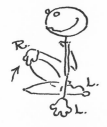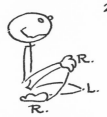

2. SHIFT BODY WEIGHT TO RELAXED LEFT ANKLE... LEAVE RIGHT TOES IN PLACE ON FLOOR... LIFT RIGHT KNEE AS HIGH AS POSSIBLE... KEEP STERNUM CENTERED OVER LEFT THIGH... HOLD ...

3. LOWER RIGHT KNEE TO FLOOR... REPEAT POSE ON OTHER SIDE, RAISING LEFT KNEE... REST IN A THUNDERBOLT POSE.

---------------------------------------------

## {ANKLE BALANCE 2}

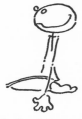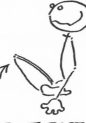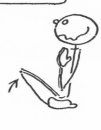

1. FROM A THUNDERBOLT POSE (P. 40)... TOUCH HANDS LIGHTLY ON FLOOR FOR BALANCE (OPPOSITE HIPS)... KEEP SPINE STRAIGHT, SHOULDERS LEVEL, FEET AND ANKLES COMPLETELY RELAXED...

2. SHIFT BODY WEIGHT TO FEET/ANKLES... LIFT KNEES AS HIGH AS POSSIBLE... KEEP KNEES TOGETHER... (TRY NOT TO LEAN BACKWARD)... FOCUS STRAIGHT AHEAD...

3. BALANCE ON RELAXED FEET... JOIN PALMS IN FRONT OF CHEST... KEEP ELBOWS CLOSE TO SIDES... HOLD ..

4. LOWER KNEES TO FLOOR, HANDS TO KNEES... REST IN A THUNDERBOLT POSE.

## { HEAD TO KNEE 2 }

1. FROM A SEATED POSE (P. 38)...
BEND RIGHT KNEE...LOWER KNEE
SIDEWAYS TO FLOOR...PULL HEEL
IN CLOSE TO GROIN...LAY SOLE
AGAINST (NOT UNDER) INNER LEFT
THIGH...KEEP RIGHT LEG RELAXED,
STERNUM IN LINE WITH
LEFT FOOT...PLACE
HANDS ON LEFT KNEE...

2. STRETCH ARMS OUT SIDEWAYS AND UP OVER HEAD..
(LET STRETCH BEGIN FROM HIPBONES TO "OPEN"
SPINE)...

3. LOOK UP BETWEEN HANDS...ARCH SPINE GENTLY
BACKWARD (KEEP CHIN LIFTED AND BACK CURVED
AS LONG AS POSSIBLE)...DO NOT ALLOW LEFT KNEE
TO BEND...

4. REACH AS FAR FORWARD AS POSSIBLE, DIRECTING
STRETCH OUT OVER (AND BEYOND) FOOT...

5. INTERLOCK FINGERS BEHIND TOES...
RELAX LEFT FOOT...PULL TOES
TOWARD BODY..(IF REACHING THE
FOOT IS AT FIRST IMPOSSIBLE, HOLD
SIDES OF ANKLE OR CALF)...
KEEP ABDOMEN RELAXED...

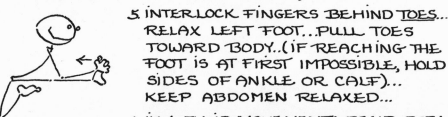

6. IN 1 FLUID MOVEMENT: BEND BOTH
ELBOWS DOWN TO FLOOR (OR BOTH
THE SAME DISTANCE FROM FLOOR)
ROLL CHEST DOWN ONTO THIGH...
RELAX NECK...GENTLY PULL TOP
OF HEAD TOWARD FOOT...[HOLD]...

7. RELEASE TOES...ROLL UP SLOWLY UNTIL SPINE
IS ERECT (SLIDING HANDS UP SHIN)...EXTEND
RIGHT LEG...REPEAT POSE (OTHER SIDE)...
REST IN A SEATED POSE.

{ TREE 2 }

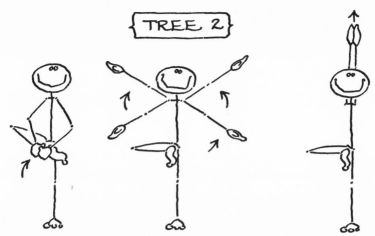

1. FROM A STANDING POSE (P 38) SEPARATE
   FEET 1 INCH APART... KEEP <u>BACK</u> <u>ERECT</u> AND
   <u>SHOULDERS</u> <u>LEVEL</u>... BEND RIGHT LEG AND
   BRING RIGHT HEEL TOWARD ABDOMEN...
   HOLD FRONT OF RIGHT ANKLE AND PLACE
   RIGHT SOLE AGAINST <u>INSIDE</u> OF LEFT
   THIGH (HEEL CLOSE TO GROIN, TOES POINTING
   DOWN)... LOCK LEFT KNEE...

2. PRESS RIGHT KNEE OUT SIDEWAYS IN LINE
   WITH RIGHT SHOULDER... KEEP CHEST
   FORWARD AND STERNUM LIFTED.. STRETCH
   ARMS OUT SIDEWAYS AND UP OVER HEAD..

3. JOIN PALMS... LOCK ELBOWS... FOCUS
   STRAIGHT AHEAD... [HOLD]...

4. STRETCH ARMS OUT SIDEWAYS AND DOWN TO
   RIGHT ANKLE... RELEASE AND LOWER FOOT...
   REPEAT POSE (OTHER SIDE) ... REST IN A
   STANDING POSE.

-----------------------------------------------

{ STAR 1 }

1. PLACE RIGHT KNEE ON TOP OF LEFT
   IN THE HEROIC POSE (P. 41)

2. LAY CHEST ON LEGS... RELAX NECK
   AND LAY CHIN OVER RIGHT KNEE...
   REST FOREARMS AND ELBOWS ON FLOOR
   NEAR LEGS (1 PALM ON TOP OF
   OTHER)... RELAX LEGS, BODY...
   [HOLD]...

3 ROLL UP SLOWLY... BRING HANDS TO
   RIGHT KNEE... REPEAT (LEFT KNEE ON TOP)...
   REST IN AN EASY POSE (P. 39 ).

## { BACK STRETCH 2 }

1. FROM A SEATED POSE (P. 38) STRETCH ARMS OUT SIDEWAYS AND UP OVER HEAD... KEEP KNEES GENTLY LOCKED...

STRAIGHT     ARCH     SOFT

2. LOOK UP BETWEEN HANDS... ARCH SPINE BACKWARD... SLOWLY REACH AS FAR FORWARD AS POSSIBLE (CHIN UP)...(STRETCH TRAVELS FROM COCCYX THROUGH → FINGER TIPS)...

3. WITHOUT LOSING ANY OF THE FORWARD STRETCH IN THE SPINE, SLIP FIRST 2 FINGERS OF EACH HAND AROUND BIG TOE (PALMS SHOULD BE FACING EACH OTHER)... (AT FIRST IT MAY BE NECESSARY TO HOLD OUTER ANKLES)...EXHALE WHILE PRESSING ELBOWS DOWN TO (OR TOWARD) FLOOR... ROLL BODY ONTO LEGS...RELAX NECK AND ABDOMEN...GENTLY, STEADILY PULL HEAD AND TOES CLOSER TOGETHER.... HOLD ... (KEEP BOTH ELBOWS THE SAME DISTANCE FROM FLOOR IF THEY WILL NOT YET TOUCH)...

4. RELEASE TOES...ROLL SPINE UP STRAIGHT (1 VERTEBRA AT A TIME), SLIDING HANDS UP SHINS... REST IN A SEATED POSE.

------------------------------------------------

## { SPINAL TWIST 3 }

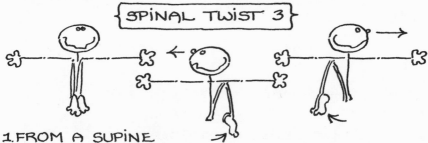

1. FROM A SUPINE POSE (P. 40)...EXTEND ARMS IN A "T" POSITION WITH PALMS DOWN...BEND LEGS...BRING KNEES TO CHEST... KEEP KNEES TOGETHER, FEET TOGETHER, AND SHOULDERS TOUCHING FLOOR....

2. SLOWLY-SMOOTHLY ROLL LEGS LEFT TO TOUCH FLOOR AND FACE RIGHT TO FOCUS BEYOND HAND... HOLD ... CENTER KNEES-FACE...REPEAT (OTHER SIDE)...REST IN A SUPINE POSE.

## {BACKWARD BEND}

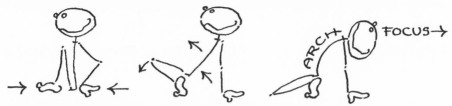

1. FROM A SEATED POSE (P 38)... BEND LEGS... PULL KNEES TOWARD CHEST... BRING HEELS AS CLOSE TO HIPS AS POSSIBLE... PLACE PALMS ON FLOOR BEHIND HIPS (FINGERS POINTING AWAY FROM BODY)... BRING WRISTS AS CLOSE TO HIPS AS POSSIBLE... KEEP HANDS IN PLACE AND KNEES TOGETHER DURING ENTIRE POSE...

2. IN 1 FLUID MOVEMENT: LIFT HIPS, THEN HEELS, AND PUSH KNEES FORWARD AND DOWN TO (OR TOWARD) FLOOR... HIPS AND HEELS WILL STAY CLOSE TOGETHER...

3. ARCH SPINE GENTLY BACKWARD, RAISING STERNUM TOWARD CEILING... RELAX NECK... LOWER HEAD... FOCUS ON REAR WALL... KEEP SHOULDERS DOWN AWAY FROM NECK... HOLD ...

4. SMOOTHLY LIFT HEAD AND KNEES... LOWER HEELS TO FLOOR, THEN HIPS... EXTEND LEGS... BRING HANDS TO KNEES... REST IN A SEATED POSE.

------------------------------------------

## {PENDANT POSE}

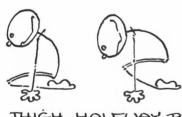

1. FROM A THUNDERBOLT POSE (P. 40) PLACE PALMS ON FLOOR (FINGERS SPREAD AND POINTING AWAY FROM LEGS... INNER WRIST TOUCHING OUTER THIGH HALFWAY BETWEEN KNEE AND HIP)...

2. LEAN FORWARD... FOCUS ON FLOOR NEAR KNEES.. RELAX NECK... LOCK ELBOW... SHIFT BODY WEIGHT FORWARD TO HANDS-ARMS... LIFT KNEES AS HIGH AS POSSIBLE (USE TOES FOR BALANCE ONLY)... HOLD ...

3. LOWER KNEES SLOWLY TO FLOOR... REST IN A THUNDERBOLT POSE.

## {POSE OF TRANQUILITY}

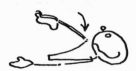

1. FROM A SUPINE POSE (P. 40) DRAW BOTH KNEES TO CHEST... KEEP ARMS CLOSE TO BODY, LEGS TOGETHER... GENTLY PRESS LUMBAR TO FLOOR...

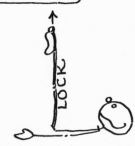

2. UNFOLD LEGS STRAIGHT UP... LOCK KNEES... POINT TOES... <u>KEEP FACE, SHOULDERS, NECK RELAXED</u>...

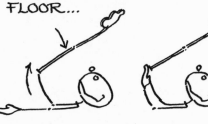

3. PRESS ARMS GENTLY AGAINST FLOOR TO LIFT HIPS OFF FLOOR... TILT LEGS BACK OVER HEAD (NO LOWER THAN 45°)... PLACE PALMS ON SACRUM..

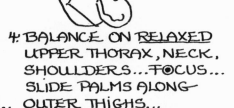

4. BALANCE ON <u>RELAXED</u> UPPER THORAX, NECK, SHOULDERS... FOCUS... SLIDE PALMS ALONG OUTER THIGHS...

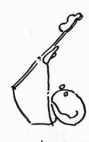

5. STRAIGHTEN ARMS... REST PALMS ON SHINS JUST BEYOND KNEES... KEEP ANGLE BETWEEN BODY AND LEGS AT LEAST 90°... (<u>NEVER TURN HEAD DURING AN INVERTED POSE</u>)... HOLD ...

6. SLIDE PALMS SLOWLY, EVENLY, ALONG OUTER THIGHS... LOWER ELBOWS, THEN PALMS, TO FLOOR (SHOULDER- WIDTH APART)... ...BEND LEGS AND LOWER KNEES TO FACE (SHINS PARALLEL TO REAR WALL)... DROP FEET BACK OVER HEAD... <u>RELAX NECK</u>... KEEP HEAD ON FLOOR, LEGS CLOSE TO BODY... ROLL SPINE DOWN SLOWLY, SMOOTHLY, I VERTEBRA AT A TIME... WHEN SACRUM TOUCHES FLOOR, BRING FEET TO FLOOR (KNEES STILL BENT).. REST IN SUPINE POSE.

{HAND TO FOOT 2}

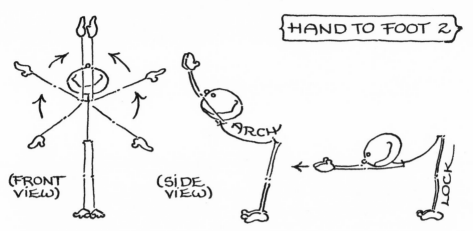

(FRONT VIEW)  (SIDE VIEW)

1. FROM A STANDING POSE (P. 38) SEPARATE FEET HIP-WIDTH APART... STRETCH ARMS SIDEWAYS AND UP OVER HEAD... LIFT CHIN (FOCUS BEYOND HANDS DURING FORWARD STRETCH)...
2. ARCH SPINE GENTLY BACKWARD... LOCK KNEES... STRETCH AND REACH AS FAR FORWARD AS POSSIBLE, THEN AS FAR DOWN AS POSSIBLE...
3. STRETCH FROM COCCYX ⟶ FINGERTIPS ⟶

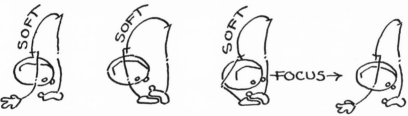

4. DEEPLY RELAX NECK, SHOULDERS, FULL LENGTH OF SPINE AND ABDOMINAL WALL (KEEP THESE AREAS SOFT!)... SHIFT WEIGHT TO HEELS...
5. FOLD EACH HAND UNDER END OF FOOT (FINGERS POINTING TOWARD HEEL)...
6. WITH UPPER BODY AND NECK RELAXED, BEND ELBOWS GENTLY OUTWARD TO PULL TOP OF HEAD TOWARD FLOOR.... (DO NOT ALLOW KNEES TO TURN INWARD)... FOCUS ON REAR WALL... HOLD ...
7. RELEASE 1 HAND AT A TIME... PAUSE... STRETCH SLOWLY FORWARD AGAIN AND UP TO CEILING... FLOAT ARMS OUT SIDEWAYS AND DOWN... REST IN A STANDING POSE.

{OPEN BOOK}

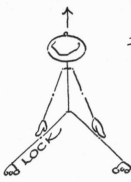

1. FROM A SPREAD FOOT POSE (P. 39)...
SEPARATE FEET 4 FEET APART...
KEEP INNER EDGES OF FEET
PARALLEL, <u>KNEES</u> <u>LOCKED</u>, <u>THIGH</u>
<u>MUSCLES TIGHT</u>, ARMS STRAIGHT
DURING ENTIRE POSE... LAY PALMS
ON OUTER THIGHS... LOOK UP...
ARCH SPINE GENTLY BACKWARD...
KEEP CHIN LIFTED...

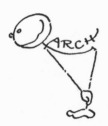

2. SLIDE PALMS DOWN OUTER LEGS
WHILE STRETCHING STERNUM AS
FAR <u>FORWARD</u> AND <u>DOWN</u> AS
POSSIBLE... KEEP SPINE ARCHED
AS LONG AS POSSIBLE (IN ORDER
TO STRETCH THE SPINE 1
VERTEBRA AT A TIME)...

 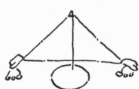

3. WHEN FULLY STRETCHED,
WRAP HANDS (ONE AT
A TIME) AROUND
BEHIND HEELS OR
ANKLES... (KEEP THUMB
WITH FINGERS)...

4. <u>GENTLY</u> PULL CENTER FRONT OF FOREHEAD TO,
OR TOWARD, FLOOR... (KEEP WEIGHT CENTERED
BETWEEN FEET AND AVOID ROLLING FORWARD
ON HEAD)... (IF ELBOWS BEND, SLIDE HANDS
FURTHER DOWN LEGS OR SPREAD FEET
FURTHER APART)... FOCUS ON FLOOR... [HOLD]...

5. KEEP THIGH MUSCLES <u>TIGHT</u>... SLOWLY STRETCH
CHEST FORWARD AND UP UNTIL BACK ERECT...
AT THE SAME TIME SLIDE PALMS UP LEGS.
REST IN A STANDING POSE (P. 38).

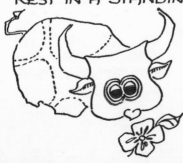

{HALF MOON 1}

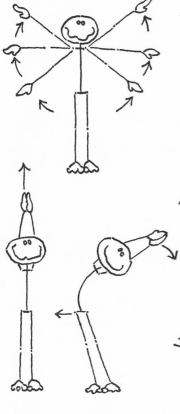

1. FROM A STANDING POSE (P. 38)... SEPARATE PARALLEL FEET HIP-DISTANCE APART... KEEP BOTH FEET ON FLOOR AND KNEES LOCKED DURING ENTIRE POSE... STRETCH ARMS SLOWLY OUT SIDEWAYS AND UP OVER HEAD...

2. JOIN PALMS, CROSS THUMBS... STRETCH UP... LOCK ELBOWS AGAINST EARS... KEEP ARMS STRAIGHT AND GENTLY STRETCHED DURING POSE... (AVOID UNNECESSARY TENSION IN SHOULDERS AND NECK)..

3. PRESS RIGHT OUTER HIP AS FAR OUT SIDEWAYS AS POSSIBLE... LEAN INTO HIP. GENTLY STRETCH ARMS LEFT..

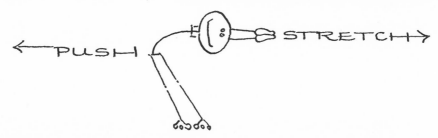

←—— PUSH        STRETCH —→

4. KEEP BOTH SHOULDERS AND BOTH HIPBONES EXACTLY SAME DISTANCE FROM FRONT WALL.... (MOVE AS IF BACK IS AGAINST A WALL)... FOCUS STRAIGHT AHEAD... [HOLD]...

5. REACH UP AGAIN SLOWLY TO STRAIGHTEN BODY... REPEAT POSE (OTHER SIDE), STRETCHING ARMS RIGHT... REST IN A STANDING POSE.

{TOE POSE 1}

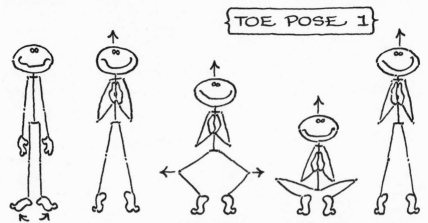

1. FROM A STANDING POSE (P. 38) SEPARATE PARALLEL FEET HIP-DISTANCE APART...TURN TOES OUT, CREATING A RIGHT ANGLE BETWEEN INNER EDGES OF FEET...

2. JOIN PALMS IN FRONT OF CHEST AND REST ELBOWS AGAINST SIDES...STRETCH TOP OF HEAD TOWARD CEILING DURING ENTIRE POSE...RISE (AND REMAIN) AS HIGH ON TOES AS POSSIBLE...FOCUS STRAIGHT AHEAD...KEEP BACK ERECT...

3. SLOWLY BEND KNEES OUTWARD (EXACTLY IN LINE WITH TOES)...KEEP SHOULDERS LEVEL...

4. LOWER BODY INTO A FULL SQUAT, KEEPING HEELS HIGH AND KNEES TURNED OUTWARD... HOLD ...

5. STRAIGHTEN LEGS IN 1 SMOOTH MOVEMENT...LOWER HEELS AND HANDS...TURN TOES FORWARD...REST IN A STANDING POSE.

-------------------------------------------------

{TOE POSE 2}

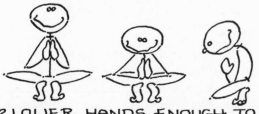

1. REPEAT STEPS 1-4 FROM ABOVE POSE... ...LEAN FORWARD AND PRESS EACH ELBOW AGAINST INNER THIGH...

2. LOWER HANDS ENOUGH TO BRING BOTH FOREARMS IN 1 LINE...WEDGE ELBOWS BETWEEN THIGHS... GENTLY SPREAD KNEES FURTHER APART WITH ELBOW PRESSURE...FOCUS ON FLOOR... HOLD ...

3. STRAIGHTEN LEGS AND BACK...LOWER HEELS AND HANDS...TURN TOES FORWARD...REST IN A STANDING POSE.

## { LORD OF DANCERS }

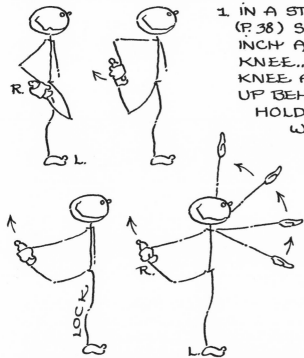

1. IN A STANDING POSE (P. 38) SEPARATE FEET 1 INCH APART...LOCK LEFT KNEE...BEND RIGHT KNEE AND BRING FOOT UP BEHIND RIGHT HIP... HOLD FRONT OF FOOT WITH RIGHT HAND (THUMB AND FINGERS TOGETHER)... KEEP RIGHT ARM AND RIGHT SHOULDER <u>RELAXED</u> DURING ENTIRE POSE...BACK SHOULD STAY <u>ERECT</u>...

2. KICK RIGHT FOOT STRAIGHT BACK-AND-UP AS FAR AS POSSIBLE (BRING OUTER RIGHT ANKLEBONE IN LINE WITH OUTER RIGHT HIP).. <u>DO</u> <u>NOT</u> <u>PULL</u> <u>ON</u> <u>RIGHT</u> <u>FOOT</u>...

3. SLOWLY STRETCH LEFT ARM FORWARD AND STRAIGHT UP OVER SHOULDER (PALM FORWARD) ...GENTLY LIFT STERNUM...

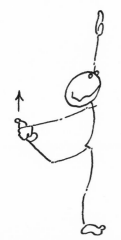

4. RAISE FACE AND FOCUS ON CEILING BEYOND LEFT HAND... HOLD ...

5. BRING LEFT ARM FORWARD AND DOWN...LOWER RIGHT KNEE...RELEASE AND LOWER RIGHT FOOT TO FLOOR... REPEAT POSE (OTHER SIDE), KICKING WITH LEFT LEG... REST IN A STANDING POSE.

## {NECK ROLL}

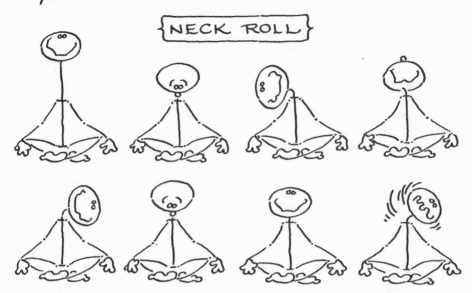

1. IN AN EASY POSE (P. 39)... KEEP BACK ERECT, STERNUM GENTLY LIFTED, NECK RELAXED, AND SHOULDERS LEVEL...

2. LAY CHIN ON CHEST... ROLL HEAD IN <u>SLOW</u> WIDE CIRCLES, FIRST RIGHT, THEN LEFT... (IN SIDE-TILT, DROP EAR OVER SHOULDER AND TURN FACE FORWARD)... ALLOW WEIGHT OF HEAD TO STRETCH NECK.

---

## {LION}

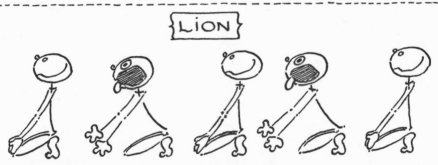

1. FROM A THUNDERBOLT POSE (P. 40)... COME UP ON TOES... INHALE DEEPLY...

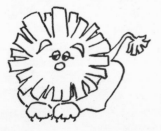

2. EXHALE AND: SLOWLY LEAN FORWARD, STRETCH ARMS, SPREAD FINGERS, WIDEN EYES, STRETCH TONGUE OUT AND DOWN... (NO HOLD)

3. SLOWLY PULL TONGUE IN AND RETURN TO A THUNDERBOLT POSE... REPEAT.

## {COWHEAD POSE 1}

1. FROM A THUNDERBOLT POSE (P. 40)... STRETCH LEFT ARM AROUND BEHIND BACK...LAY BACK OF LEFT HAND AS HIGH ON SPINE AS POSSIBLE...KEEP <u>HIPS</u> <u>ON</u> <u>HEELS</u> AND SPINE STRAIGHT...

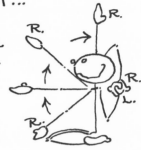

2. SLOWLY STRETCH RIGHT ARM FORWARD AND UP OVER HEAD...BEND RIGHT ELBOW... REACH DOWN WITH RIGHT HAND...HOOK FINGERS OF BOTH HANDS TOGETHER (AT FIRST IT MAY BE NECESSARY TO HOLD A SMALL TOWEL TO LINK HANDS)... CURL FINGERS TIGHTLY TO PULL RIGHT ARM BEHIND HEAD... (DO NOT ALLOW HEAD TO TILT AND <u>KEEP</u> <u>SHOULDERS</u> <u>RELAXED</u>)...

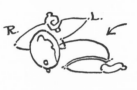

3. STRETCH UPPER BODY FORWARD AND ROLL CHEST DOWN ONTO THIGHS...BRING FOREHEAD TO FLOOR (WITHOUT LIFTING OFF OF HEELS)... [HOLD]...

4. STRETCH UPPER BODY FORWARD AGAIN... STRAIGHTEN BACK...UNLOCK FINGERS.... RETURN HANDS TO KNEES...REPEAT POSE ON OTHER SIDE... REST IN THUNDERBOLT POSE.

---

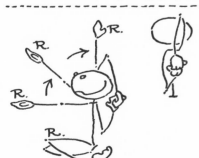

## {COWHEAD POSE 2}

VARIATION: PRACTICE POSE AS DESCRIBED ABOVE, BUT WITH LEGS FOLDED IN THE HEROIC POSE (P. 41)... PLACE <u>RIGHT</u> KNEE ON TOP WHEN <u>RIGHT</u> ARM IS OVER HEAD-LEFT KNEE ON TOP WHEN LEFT ARM IS OVER HEAD.

## { HALF LOTUS }

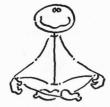 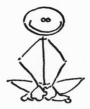 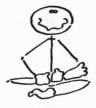 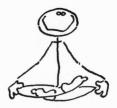

1. FROM AN EASY POSE (P. 39) WITH LEFT HEEL CLOSE TO GROIN... <u>KEEP BACK ERECT</u> AND <u>HIPS, LEGS, ANKLES, FEET DEEPLY RELAXED</u>...

2. HOLD FRONT OF RIGHT ANKLE (NOT FOOT OR TOES)... BEND ELBOWS TO LIFT FOOT AND PULL RIGHT HEEL TOWARD NAVEL... LAY OUTER FOOT AND ANKLE (NOT JUST TOES) ACROSS UPPER LEFT THIGH (AS CLOSE TO ABDOMEN AS POSSIBLE).. FOCUS STRAIGHT AHEAD...

3. RELEASE ANKLE... REST HANDS ON KNEES... HOLD ... CAREFULLY SLIDE RIGHT FOOT OFF LEFT LEG... REPEAT POSE (OTHER SIDE).. REST IN A SEATED POSE (P. 38).

-------------------------------------------------

## { GENTLE POSE }

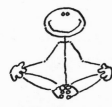 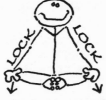 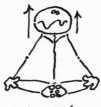 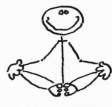

1. FROM A SEATED POSE (P. 38) BRING HEELS CLOSE TO GROIN... TURN SOLES OF FEET TOGETHER... ALLOW KNEES TO DROP OUT SIDEWAYS... <u>KEEP BACK ERECT</u> (AT FIRST IT MAY BE HELPFUL TO PLACE THE BACK AGAINST A WALL)...

2. CUP HANDS OVER ENDS OF KNEES (FINGERS SPREAD)... RELAX SHOULDERS... PRESS KNEES TO FLOOR IN ① <u>STEADY PUSH</u>, WHILE LOCKING ELBOWS (SHOULDER GIRDLE WILL BE LIFTED OFF UPPER RIBCAGE)... WEDGE STRAIGHT ARMS BETWEEN KNEES AND RAISED SHOULDERS... KEEP LEGS AND HIPS COMPLETELY RELAXED... FOCUS STRAIGHT AHEAD AND HOLD ...

3. RELAX ARMS... REST IN A SEATED POSE (P. 38).

## { STANDING BOW }

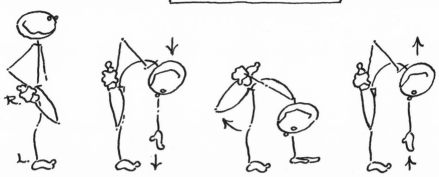

1. SEPARATE PARALLEL FEET 1 INCH IN A STANDING POSE (P. 38)... BRING RIGHT HEEL UP TO TOUCH RIGHT BUTTOCK... HOLD RIGHT ANKLE WITH RIGHT HAND... (HEEL TOUCHES HIP DURING ENTIRE POSE)... LOCK LEFT KNEE...

2. FOCUS ON FLOOR ABOUT 12 INCHES IN FRONT OF LEFT FOOT... LEAN DOWN SLOOOOWLY AND TOUCH HAND ON FLOOR (IN LINE WITH LEFT SHOULDER), WHILE SWINGING RIGHT KNEE STRAIGHT BACK... (DO NOT SWING KNEE OUT SIDEWAYS)...

3. LEFT ARM SHOULD BE PERPENDICULAR TO FLOOR... USE LEFT HAND FOR BALANCE ONLY... HOLD ...

4. RAISE UP SLOWLY... RELEASE AND LOWER RIGHT FOOT... REPEAT POSE (OTHER SIDE), BENDING LEFT LEG... REST IN A STANDING POSE.

- - - - - - - - - - - - - - - - - - - - - - - - - - - - - - - - - - -

## { COBBLER }

1. FROM AN EASY POSE (P. 39) TURN SOLES OF FEET TOGETHER... BRING HEELS CLOSE TO GROIN...

2. INTERLOCK FINGERS AROUND TOES... KEEP SHOULDERS DOWN, HIPS ON FLOOR, ELBOWS CLOSE TO HIPS...

3. PULL AGAINST TOES TO STRETCH STERNUM FORWARD AND DOWN TO TOUCH FEET... RELAX NECK... LAY FACE ON FLOOR... HOLD ...

4. REST CHIN ON CHEST... ROLL SPINE SLOWLY UP STRAIGHT... REST IN AN EASY POSE.

## {SMALL BOAT}

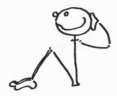 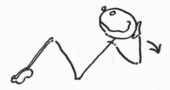

1. FROM A SEATED POSE (P. 38)... KEEP LEGS AND FEET TOGETHER, SPINE STRAIGHT, <u>STERNUM LIFTED</u> DURING POSE... BEND KNEES...

2. LACE FINGERS TOGETHER BEHIND HEAD (FIT THUMBS IN HOLLOW AT BASE OF SKULL)... KEEP ELBOWS COMFORTABLY SPREAD... TILT BACK...

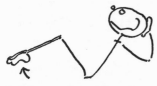 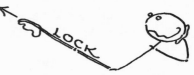

3. BALANCE BETWEEN SACRUM AND COCCYX... LIFT TOES OFF FLOOR... TILT SPINE AT A 30° ANGLE WITH FLOOR...

4. UNFOLD LEGS (ALSO AT A 30° ANGLE)... LOCK KNEES... POINT TOES... KEEP TOP OF HEAD IN LINE WITH TOES... FOCUS OVER TOES... HOLD ...

5. BEND KNEES... LOWER FEET TO FLOOR... STRAIGHTEN BACK... BRING HANDS TO KNEES... REST IN A SEATED POSE.

- - - - - - - - - - - - - - - - - - - - - - - - - - - - - - - - - - -

## {UPWARD LEG STRETCH}

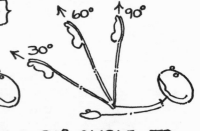

1. FROM A SUPINE POSE (P. 40) KEEP LEGS TOGETHER... BEND LEGS... DRAW KNEES TO CHEST...

2. <u>SLOWLY</u> UNFOLD LEGS AT A 30° ANGLE TO FLOOR... LOCK KNEES, POINT TOES... KEEP SACRUM CLOSE FLOOR... FOCUS STRAIGHT UP... HOLD ... BEND LEGS... DRAW KNEES TO CHEST...

3. REPEAT STEP #2 AT 60°, THEN 90°...

4. WITH KNEES BENT, PLACE FEET ON FLOOR... EXTEND LEGS... REST IN A SUPINE POSE.

## {RIGHT ANGLE POSE}

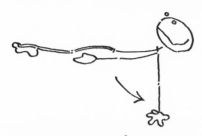 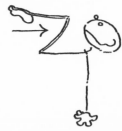

1. FROM A SUPINE POSE (P. 40) EXTEND ARMS SIDEWAYS AT SHOULDER-LEVEL, PALMS DOWN

2. BEND LEGS AND PULL KNEES TO CHEST... PRESS SACRUM TO FLOOR...

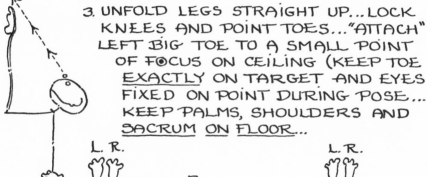

3. UNFOLD LEGS STRAIGHT UP... LOCK KNEES AND POINT TOES... "ATTACH" LEFT BIG TOE TO A SMALL POINT OF FOCUS ON CEILING (KEEP TOE EXACTLY ON TARGET AND EYES FIXED ON POINT DURING POSE... KEEP PALMS, SHOULDERS AND SACRUM ON FLOOR...

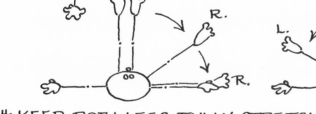 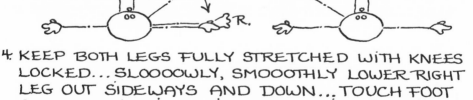

4. KEEP BOTH LEGS FULLY STRETCHED WITH KNEES LOCKED... SLOOOOWLY, SMOOOTHLY LOWER RIGHT LEG OUT SIDEWAYS AND DOWN... TOUCH FOOT ON FLOOR IN LINE WITH OUTER HIP...[HOLD]...

5. SLOOOWLY RAISE RIGHT LEG STRAIGHT UP... REPEAT POSE (OTHER SIDE), LOWERING LEFT LEG. REST IN A SUPINE POSE.

## { HEAD TO KNEE 5 }

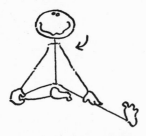
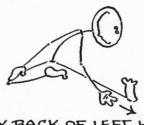

1. FROM A SEATED POSE (P.38)...BEND RIGHT KNEE...BRING RIGHT HEEL CLOSE TO GROIN BUT KEEP FOOT OUT FROM UNDER LEFT THIGH...REST RIGHT KNEE ON FLOOR...TURN CHEST TOWARD RIGHT KNEE...

2. LAY BACK OF LEFT HAND ON FLOOR INSIDE (AND NEAR) LEFT LEG...LOOK BEYOND RIGHT KNEE... SLIDE LEFT HAND ALONG FLOOR (CLOSE TO LEG) AS FAR AS POSSIBLE... RELAX NECK...LAY LEFT EAR ON SHOULDER... RELAX WAIST MUSCLES...

3. STRETCH RIGHT ARM SLOWLY UP OVER HEAD, TOWARD LEFT FOOT... RIGHT ARM MUST PASS EXACTLY OVER EAR... (RIGHT DOES NOT DROP IN FRONT OF FACE)...KEEP CHEST TURNED TOWARD RIGHT KNEE...

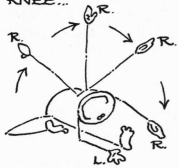

4. INTERLOCK FINGERS BEHIND LEFT HEEL (THUMBS ON FLOOR)... GENTLY BEND BOTH ELBOWS TO PULL HEAD TOWARD LEFT FOOT...PRESS LEFT ELBOW TO FLOOR... KEEP NECK RELAXED... HOLD

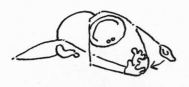

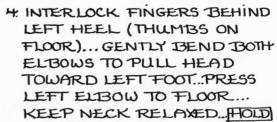

5. RELEASE FOOT... STRETCH RIGHT ARM OVER HEAD...REST RIGHT HAND ON RIGHT KNEE... ROLL UP SLOWLY UNTIL BACK ERECT...REPEAT POSE (OTHER SIDE)...REST IN A SEATED POSE.

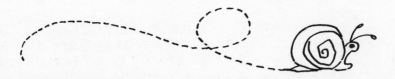

{ DOG, FACE TO THE MOON }

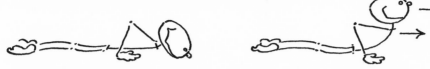

1. FROM A PRONE POSE (P. 38) SEPARATE FEET HIP-WIDTH APART... POINT TOES... PLACE PALMS ON FLOOR, CLOSE TO BODY (FINGERS POINTING TOWARD HEAD AND BEND OF WRIST AT WAIST)...

2. IN 1 FLUID MOVEMENT: STRETCH AND LENGTHEN SPINE... LIFT FACE, THEN CHEST (STRETCH FORWARD AS WELL AS UP)...

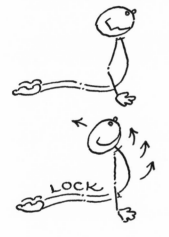

3. SLOWLY STRAIGHTEN ARMS... LOCK ELBOWS... KEEP NECK LONG AND OPEN, <u>SHOULDERS DOWN</u>...

4. LOCK KNEES TO RAISE LEGS A SMALL DISTANCE FROM FLOOR...BALANCE ON PALMS AND FRONTS OF FEET..PUSH STERNUM GENTLY FORWARD AND FOCUS STRAIGHT UP... HOLD ...

5. LOWER LEGS...BEND ELBOWS BACKWARD TO ROLL CHEST-AND-FACE FORWARD AND DOWN...REST IN PRONE POSE.

-----

{ FISH }

1. FROM A SUPINE POSE (P. 40) KEEP LEGS TOGETHER...TUCK HANDS UNDER OUTER THIGHS... ARMS STRAIGHT...PALMS DOWN...

2. PRESS ELBOWS AGAINST FLOOR TO ARCH AND RAISE SPINE...REST ON HIPS AND TOP OF HEAD...FOCUS ON REAR WALL...

3. FREE HANDS, 1 AT A TIME...REST PALMS ON FRONTS OF THIGHS... <u>KEEP</u> <u>ARCH</u> <u>HIGH</u>... HOLD ...

4. BRACE ELBOWS ON FLOOR, HOLDING OUTER THIGHS...SLIDE BACK OF HEAD TO FLOOR...LOWER BACK...REST IN A SUPINE POSE.

## {MONKEY}

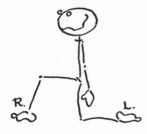

1. FROM A KNEELING POSE (P. 40) SLIDE RIGHT FOOT FORWARD (KNEE BENT, FOOT IN LINE WITH RIGHT HIP, TOES POINTING STRAIGHT AHEAD)... PUSH FRONT OF ANKLE ABOUT 5 INCHES FURTHER FORWARD THAN FRONT OF KNEE...

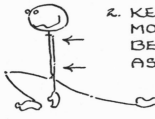

2. KEEP SPINE ERECT, ARMS DOWN... MOVE BODY FORWARD BY BENDING RIGHT KNEE AS MUCH AS POSSIBLE (WITHOUT LIFTING RIGHT HEEL OFF FLOOR)... KEEP LEFT KNEE AND TOP OF LEFT FOOT ON FLOOR...

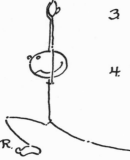

3. SLOWLY STRETCH ARMS OUT SIDEWAYS AND UP OVER HEAD... JOIN PALMS... LOCK ELBOWS...

4. ARCH SPINE BACKWARD... SLOWLY STRETCH ARMS AS FAR BACK AS POSSIBLE... KEEP EARS BETWEEN UPPER ARMS AND FOCUS ON CEILING... [HOLD]...

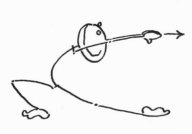

5. REACH FOR CEILING AGAIN TO STRAIGHTEN BACK... FLOAT ARMS OUT SIDEWAYS AND DOWN... RETURN TO A KNEELING POSE AND REPEAT ENTIRE POSE (OTHER SIDE)... REST IN A THUNDERBOLT POSE.

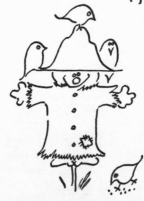

## { PLOUGH }

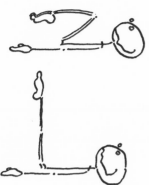

1. FROM A SUPINE POSE (P. 40), TUCK ARMS IN CLOSE TO BODY, PALMS DOWN... GENTLY STRETCH ARMS TO PULL SHOULDERS AWAY FROM NECK... DRAW BENT KNEES TO CHEST... KEEP LEGS TOGETHER..

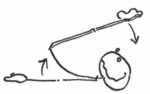

2. PRESS SACRUM TO FLOOR... SLOWLY UNFOLD LEGS STRAIGHT UP... LOCK KNEES AND POINT TOES... REMAIN IN THIS POSITION ABOUT 30 SECONDS...

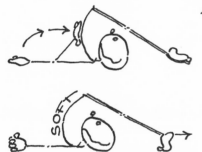

3. GENTLY PRESS FULL LENGTH OF ARMS AGAINST FLOOR... IN 1 FLUID MOVEMENT: RAISE HIPS UP OFF FLOOR AND TILT LOCKED LEGS OVER BODY/HEAD

4. RELAX ENTIRE SPINE AND ALLOW GRAVITY TO LOWER FEET TO FLOOR... BEND ARMS AND BRACE PALMS ON BACK... KEEP ELBOWS NO MORE THAN SHOULDER-WIDTH APART... DO NOT TURN HEAD OR TUCK CHIN DOWN... FOCUS...

5. TURN TOES UNDER... CAREFULLY LOWER ARMS TO FLOOR AND INTERLOCK FINGERS... LOCK ELBOWS AND BRING INNER WRISTS TOGETHER... RELAX FROM BASE OF SKULL TO COCCYX... PUSH HEELS GENTLY AWAY FROM HEAD... HOLD ...

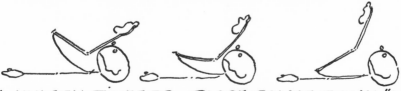

6. UNLOCK FINGERS... PLACE PALMS DOWN... "WALK" TOES TOWARD HEAD... BEND KNEES (KEEP THIGHS CLOSE TO CHEST AND FEET OVER FACE)... RELAX NECK AND KEEP HEAD ON FLOOR... SLOWLY ROLL SPINE TO FLOOR... LOWER FEET TO FLOOR (KNEES BENT)... EXTEND LEGS... REST IN A SUPINE POSE.

{ TRIANGLE 2 }

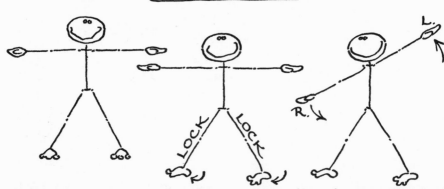

1. FROM A SPREAD FOOT POSE (P. 39) SEPARATE FEET 3 FEET APART... STRETCH ARMS OUT SIDEWAYS, LEVEL WITH FLOOR.... KEEP ARMS IN A STRAIGHT LINE DURING ENTIRE POSE...

2. TURN RIGHT ON HEELS INTO AN ANGLED FOOT POSE (P.41)... LOCK KNEES AND KEEP BOTH FEET FLAT ON FLOOR...

3. TILT STRAIGHT ARMS (AS IF LEFT HAND WERE TRACING A RAINBOW HIGH OVER HEAD)...

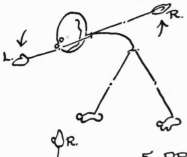

4. STRETCH LEFT HAND TOWARD END WALL, THEN TO FLOOR OUTSIDE RIGHT FOOT (OR TO RIGHT SHIN).. TWIST SPINE TO TURN CHEST TOWARD REAR WALL...(DO NOT LEAN ON LEFT HAND)...

5. BRING LEFT SHOULDER OVER RIGHT SHIN... LENGTHEN SPINE (ESPECIALLY NECK)... STRETCH RIGHT ARM STRAIGHT UP (PALM TURNED TOWARD REAR WALL)... FOCUS ON CEILING BEYOND THUMB... CONTINUE TO STRETCH SPINE... [HOLD]...

6. KEEP ARMS IN 1 LINE... RETRACE "RAINBOW" OVER HEAD WITH LEFT HAND UNTIL ARMS ARE LEVEL... TURN BODY AND FEET FORWARD... REPEAT POSE (OTHER SIDE)... REST IN A STANDING POSE (P. 38 ).

## {HALF SQUAT ON 1 LEG}

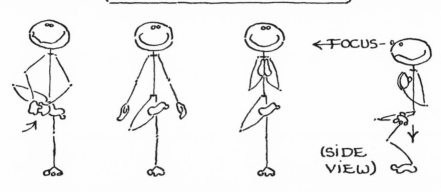

←FOCUS—

(SIDE VIEW)

1. FROM A STANDING POSE (P. 38) SEPARATE FEET 1 INCH...BEND AND RAISE RIGHT KNEE,...HOLD FRONT OF RIGHT <u>ANKLE</u> WITH BOTH HANDS... PLACE OUTER EDGE OF RIGHT FOOT ACROSS FRONT OF LEFT THIGH CLOSE TO HIP...

2. KEEP <u>BACK ERECT</u> AND <u>SHOULDERS LEVEL</u> DURING ENTIRE POSE...PRESS RIGHT KNEE GENTLY DOWN AND BACK...

3. JOIN PALMS IN FRONT OF CHEST...REST ELBOWS AGAINST SIDES...FOCUS STRAIGHT AHEAD...

4. BEND LEFT KNEE AS DEEPLY AS POSSIBLE, KEEPING HEEL ON FLOOR... HOLD ...

5. STRAIGHTEN LEFT LEG... LOWER HANDS TO RELEASE ANKLE... SLOWLY STRAIGHTEN RIGHT LEG...REPEAT POSE (OTHER SIDE), STANDING ON RIGHT FOOT... REST IN A STANDING POSE.

-----------------------------------------

## {NECK STRETCH}

1. FROM A THUNDERBOLT POSE (P. 40)... <u>KEEP BACK ERECT</u> AND <u>STERNUM LIFTED</u> DURING POSE... RELAX NECK...DROP CHIN TO CHEST...

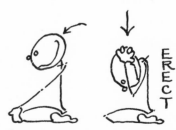

E R E C T

2. INTERLOCK FINGERS BEHIND SKULL... <u>RELAX ARMS, NECK, SHOULDERS COMPLETELY</u>...ALLOW WEIGHT OF <u>RELAXED</u> ARMS TO STRETCH NECK (DO NOT PULL HEAD DOWN !!!! ARMS MUST BE PASSIVE)...FOCUS AND HOLD ...

3. RETURN HANDS TO KNEES...REST IN A THUNDERBOLT POSE.

## { HEAD TO KNEE 6 }

1. FROM A STANDING POSE (P. 38) SEPARATE PARALLEL FEET 1 INCH APART... KEEP SPINE ERECT AND SHOULDERS LEVEL WHILE BRINGING BENT RIGHT KNEE TOWARD CHEST... <u>LOCK STANDING KNEE</u> DURING ENTIRE POSE...

2. INTERLOCK FINGERS BEHIND <u>TOES</u>...

3. SLOWLY UNFOLD RIGHT LEG FORWARD (PARALLEL TO FLOOR)... LOCK RIGHT KNEE AND PULL TOES <u>TOWARD</u> BODY...

4. IN 1 SMOOTH MOVEMENT: BEND ELBOWS DOWNWARD, PULL FACE TO RIGHT LEG, RELAX NECK... FOCUS ON FLOOR BEYOND INNER KNEE... [HOLD]...

5. BEND RIGHT KNEE... STRAIGHTEN BACK... RELEASE RIGHT FOOT AND LOWER LEG... REPEAT POSE (OTHER SIDE)... REST IN A STANDING POSE.

------

## { FULL LOCUST }

1. FROM A PRONE POSE (P. 38) POINT TOES... LOCK KNEES... KEEP LEGS TOGETHER...

2. ARCH BACK... LIFT LEGS AND CHEST (REST ON ABDOMEN BETWEEN HIPBONES AND BOTTOM RIBS)... TOES WILL BE HIGHER THAN HEAD... REACH STRAIGHT BACK (ARMS LEVEL)... FOCUS STRAIGHT AHEAD (AVOID NECK TENSION)... [HOLD]...

3. RELAX INTO A PRONE POSE. REST.

## {HERON}

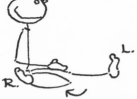 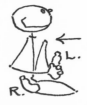

1. FROM A SEATED POSE (P.38) FOLD RIGHT LEG BACKWARD...PLACE INNER EDGE OF RIGHT FOOT ALONG CURVE OF OUTER RIGHT HIP... KEEP KNEES TOGETHER...(DO NOT SIT ON FOOT)...

2. BEND LEFT LEG AND BRING LEFT KNEE TOWARD CHEST... INTERLOCK FINGERS BEHIND LEFT HEEL... SIT STRAIGHT...

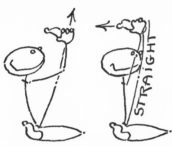

3 SLOWLY UNFOLD LEFT LEG STRAIGHT UP...LOCK KNEE..

4. SLOWLY BEND ELBOWS OUTWARD TO BRING FACE AND LEG TOGETHER..FOCUS PAST INNER LEFT KNEE... HOLD ...

5. BEND LEFT KNEE, RELEASE HEEL, EXTEND LEG... UNFOLD AND STRAIGHTEN RIGHT LEG... REPEAT POSE (OTHER SIDE), FOLDING LEFT LEG BACK...REST IN A SEATED POSE.

-----------------------------------------

## {RAISED THUNDERBOLT}

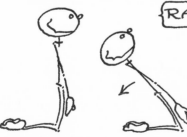

1. FROM A KNEELING POSE (P. 40) SEPARATE KNEES HIP-WIDTH APART...BRING TIPS OF BIG TOES TOGETHER...PLACE PALMS ON FRONT OF THIGHS...

2. KEEP NECK AND SPINE STRAIGHT DURING ENTIRE POSE... TILT BACKWARD AND LOWER BODY HALFWAY TO FLOOR (DO NOT RELAX NECK)...FOCUS ON CEILING... HOLD ...

3 SLOWLY RETURN TO A KNEELING POSE... REST IN A THUNDERBOLT POSE (P. 40 ).

## { 3 LIMBS }

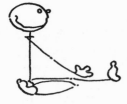

1. FROM A SEATED POSE (P. 38) FOLD RIGHT LEG BACKWARD... PLACE INNER EDGE OF RIGHT FOOT CLOSE TO CURVE OF OUTER RIGHT HIP... KEEP INNER THIGHS TOGETHER DURING POSE...

2. STRETCH ARMS OUT SIDEWAYS AND UP OVER HEAD... LIFT CHIN... GENTLY ARCH SPINE BACKWARD... SLOWLY STRETCH AS FAR BEYOND LEFT FOOT AS POSSIBLE (STRETCH SPINE AS WELL AS ARMS)...

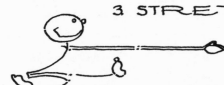

3. STRETCH → AND KEEP CHIN AND STERNUM GENTLY LIFTED AS LONG AS POSSIBLE...

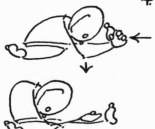

4. INTERLOCK FINGERS BEHIND HEEL (OR HOLD ANKLE)... IN 1 FLUID MOVEMENT: ROLL CHEST DOWN ONTO THIGH, RELAX NECK, PRESS ELBOWS TO (OR TOWARD) FLOOR... PULL TOP OF HEAD TOWARD FOOT... HOLD ...

5. RELEASE HEEL... ROLL SPINE UP SLOWLY UNTIL BACK IS ERECT (SLIDING THUMBS UP SHIN)... CAREFULLY UNFOLD AND EXTEND RIGHT LEG... REPEAT POSE (OTHER SIDE), FOLDING LEFT LEG BACKWARD... REST IN A SEATED POSE.

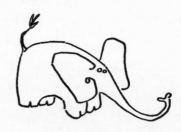

## { SPINAL TWIST 5 }

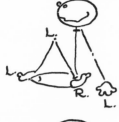

1. FROM A SEATED POSE (P. 38) BEND LEGS...DRAW KNEES TOWARD CHEST...SLIDE RIGHT FOOT AND LEG UNDER LEFT LEG-BRIDGE...PULL RIGHT HEEL AROUND TO TOUCH OUTER LEFT HIP...REST RIGHT KNEE ON FLOOR IN FRONT OF STERNUM... STEP OVER RIGHT KNEE WITH LEFT FOOT (PLACE FOOT ON FLOOR WITH OUTER LEFT ANKLEBONE TOUCHING OUTER RIGHT KNEE)...

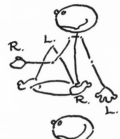

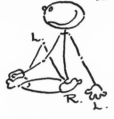

2. SLIP RIGHT ELBOW OVER LEFT KNEE...PRESS UPPER ARM AGAINST <u>OUTER</u> LEFT KNEE...

3. HOLD INNER EDGE OF <u>LEFT</u> FOOT WITH <u>RIGHT</u> HAND (OR HOLD RIGHT KNEE WITH RIGHT HAND)...KEEP SHOULDERS DOWN..

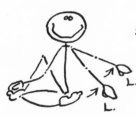

4. STRETCH LEFT ARM AROUND BEHIND BACK...HOLD INNER RIGHT THIGH WITH LEFT HAND (OR LAY BACK OF HAND ON HIP).. SIT EVENLY ON BOTH HIPS...

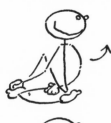

5. DURING ENTIRE POSE SIT <u>VERY</u> <u>STRAIGHT</u> AND <u>VERY</u> <u>TALL</u>.. TURN AND TWIST BODY AS FAR LEFT AS POSSIBLE (TWIST FULL LENGTH OF SPINE)...PRESS RIGHT ARM AGAINST LEFT <u>LEG</u>... FOCUS ON REAR WALL... | HOLD |...

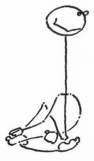

6. RELEASE FOOT AND THIGH... SLIP RIGHT ARM OVER LEFT KNEE... SWING LEFT HAND AROUND TO RIGHT KNEE...TURN FACE-CHEST FORWARD...UNFOLD LEGS...REPEAT POSE ON OTHER SIDE, TWISTING RIGHT →.

{BOW 2}

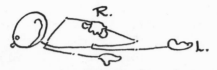

1. FROM A PRONE POSE (P.38) BEND RIGHT KNEE
   AND BRING RIGHT HEEL TO RIGHT HIP...HOLD
   FRONT OF RIGHT FOOT WITH RIGHT HAND
   (KEEP THUMB AND FINGERS TOGETHER)

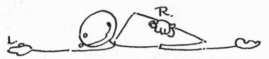

2. EXTEND LEFT ARM IN FRONT OF BODY (PALM
   DOWN AND IN LINE WITH LEFT SHOULDER)...
   KEEP RIGHT ARM AND BACK COMPLETELY
   RELAXED...

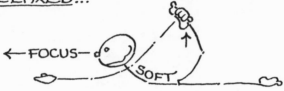

3. KEEP LEFT ARM AND FRONT OF LEFT LEG ON
   FLOOR... SMOOTHLY KICK RIGHT FOOT STRAIGHT
   UP (ALLOW THRUST OF KICK TO RAISE UPPER
   BODY...DO NOT PULL ON FOOT)...RAISE FACE
   JUST ENOUGH TO FOCUS STRAIGHT AHEAD
   (KEEP NECK RELAXED)... [HOLD]...

4. LOWER LEG, RELEASE FOOT AND STRAIGHTEN
   LEG...REPEAT POSE (OTHER SIDE), KICKING
   LEFT LEG...REST IN PRONE POSE.

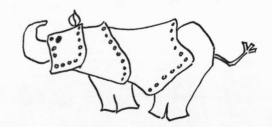

## {CAMEL 2}

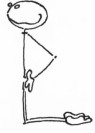 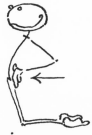 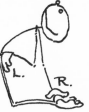 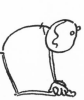

1. FROM A KNEELING POSE (P. 40) SEPARATE FEET AND LEGS HIP-WIDTH APART...PLACE HANDS ON BUTTOCKS (FINGERS SPREAD)...RELAX HIPS AND SPINE...(SWALLOW NOW, RATHER THAN DURING POSE)...

2. STEADILY PUSH HIPS-THIGHS AS FAR FORWARD AS POSSIBLE, USING HAND PRESSURE...

3. KEEP HIPS FORWARD...REACH BACK (1 HAND AT A TIME) AND GRASP FIRMLY EACH HEEL...

4. RELAX NECK AND SLOWLY LOWER HEAD...LOCK ELBOWS...KEEP SHOULDERS DOWN AND STERNUM GENTLY LIFTED...

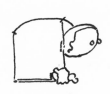

5. CREATE A SQUARE-SHAPED SPACE WITHIN LEGS-ARMS-BACK...KEEP NECK DEEPLY RELAXED...PUSH SHOULDERS GENTLY TOWARD HIPS...FOCUS ON REAR WALL...HOLD...

6. IN 1 FLUID MOVEMENT: KEEP NECK SOFT, SHIFT WEIGHT TO RIGHT HAND (OR LEFT)...RELEASE OPPOSITE HEEL AND TILT SLOWLY RIGHT, ROLLING HEAD...RELEASE RIGHT HEEL AND RETURN TO A KNEELING POSE...REST IN A THUNDERBOLT POSE (CHIN ON CHEST).

## { KNEE TO EAR }

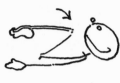

1. FROM A SUPINE POSE (P. 40) TUCK ARMS IN CLOSE TO BODY, PALMS DOWN... GENTLY STRETCH ARMS TO PULL SHOULDERS AWAY FROM NECK... DRAW BENT KNEES TO CHEST (LEGS TOGETHER)...

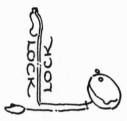

2. UNFOLD LEGS STRAIGHT UP... LOCK KNEES AND POINT TOES... REMAIN IN THIS POSITION AT LEAST 30 SECONDS...

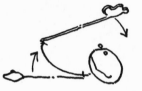

3. GENTLY PRESS FULL LENGTH OF ARMS AGAINST FLOOR... IN 1 FLUID MOVEMENT: RAISE HIPS TOWARD CEILING AND TILT LEGS OVER BODY... RELAX BACK AND NECK...

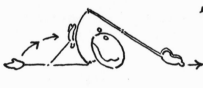

4. ALLOW GRAVITY TO PULL FEET TO FLOOR BEYOND TOP OF HEAD... BEND ARMS AND BRACE PALMS ON BACK... KEEP ELBOWS SHOULDER-WIDTH APART. CONTINUE TO RELAX FACE, NECK, ABDOMEN, AND BACK... FOCUS...

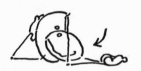

5. KEEP TIPS OF BIG TOES TOGETHER... SEPARATE KNEES... SLOWLY DRAW KNEES IN TO REST ON FLOOR CLOSE TO EARS (THIGHS SHOULD BE VERTICAL)... DO NOT FORCE KNEES DOWN... BREATHE EVENLY.. HOLD ...LOCK KNEES AGAIN...

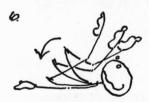

6. LOWER PALMS TO FLOOR (SHOULDER-WIDTH APART)... KEEP NECK SOFT AND HEAD ON FLOOR... ROLL SPINE DOWN ONTO FLOOR 1 VERTEBRA AT A TIME (WITH KNEES BENT, THIGHS CLOSE TO CHEST, AND FEET OVER FACE)... WHEN SACRUM TOUCHS FLOOR, BRING FEET TO FLOOR ALSO... EXTEND LEGS... REST IN A SUPINE POSE.

{ POWERFUL POSE }

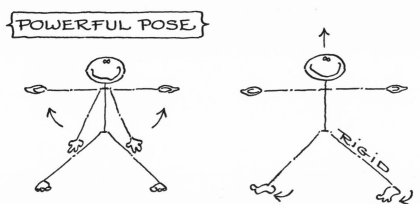

1. FROM A SPREAD FOOT POSE (P. 39) (USING A 4 FOOT SEPARATION BETWEEN FEET)... STRETCH ARMS OUT SIDEWAYS, LEVEL WITH FLOOR...

2. TURN TOES RIGHT (PIVOT ON BOTH HEELS) INTO AN ANGLED FOOT POSE (P. 41)... KEEP <u>LEFT KNEE LOCKED</u> AND ENTIRE <u>LEFT</u> <u>SOLE</u> <u>ON FLOOR</u> DURING COMPLETE POSE... STRETCH SPINE UPWARD...

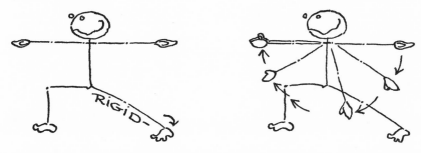

3 BEND RIGHT KNEE, CREATING A 90° ANGLE (KEEP SHIN <u>VERTICAL</u> AND THIGH LEVEL, KNEE IN LINE WITH RIGHT TOES)... FOCUS ON WALL BEYOND TOES...

4. IN 1 FLUID MOVEMENT: SLOWLY TWIST SHOULDERS RIGHT, STRETCH LEFT ARM DOWN, AND THEN UP, TO JOIN PALMS IN LINE WITH RIGHT KNEE...

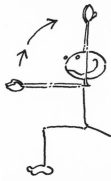

5. <u>STRETCH</u> HANDS TO CEILING OVER HEAD (KEEP NECK RELAXED)... BREATHE EVENLY... [HOLD]...

6. FLOAT ARMS OUT SIDEWAYS AND DOWN BESIDE HIPS... STRAIGHTEN RIGHT LEG... TURN TOES, BODY, FACE FORWARD... RELAX SHOULDERS... REPEAT POSE (OTHER SIDE), TURNING LEFT... REST IN A STANDING POSE (P. 38).

## {LATERAL ANGLE STRETCH}

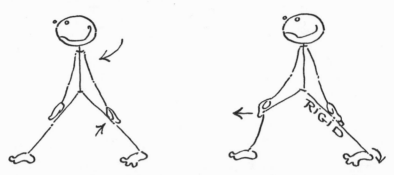

1. FROM AN ANGLED FOOT POSE (P. 41 , USING A 4 FOOT SEPARATION BETWEEN HEELS)... TURN UPPER BODY RIGHT...LAY RIGHT PALM ON FRONT OF RIGHT THIGH, LEFT PALM ON BACK OF LEFT THIGH... <u>LOCK LEFT KNEE AND KEEP IT TIGHTLY LOCKED DURING POSE</u>...PRESS <u>ENTIRE</u> SOLE OF LEFT FOOT <u>FIRMLY</u> AGAINST FLOOR...DO NOT LEAN ON RIGHT HAND...

2. KEEP LEFT LEG RIGIDLY LOCKED, WHILE SLOWLY BENDING RIGHT KNEE AND SLIDING RIGHT HAND TO FLOOR NEAR OUTER EDGE OF FOOT... LEAN FORWARD, BRINGING CHEST NEAR LEG... CREATE A RIGHT ANGLE BEHIND RIGHT KNEE (<u>THIGH LEVEL WITH FLOOR, SHIN VERTICAL</u>)...

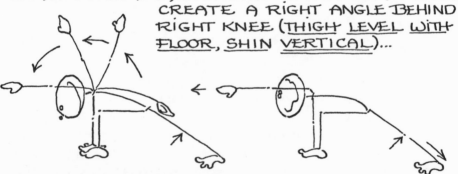

3. STRETCH LEFT ARM SLOWLY UP OVER BODY, THEN OVER HEAD (LEVEL WITH FLOOR AND IN LINE WITH RIGHT FOOT)...PULL HEAD BACKWARD, OUT FROM UNDER ARM...TURN CHEST FORWARD...

4. FOCUS ON END WALL BEYOND LEFT HAND... SPINE SHOULD BE ARCHED GENTLY BACKWARD... KEEP RIGHT KNEE IN LINE WITH TOES...|HOLD|...

5. RETURN LEFT PALM TO LEFT THIGH...SLIDE RIGHT HAND UP RIGHT LEG WHILE STRAIGHTENING KNEE... TURN TOES AND BODY FORWARD...REPEAT POSE (OTHER SIDE)...REST IN A STANDING POSE.

# { FULL LOTUS }

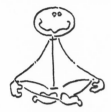

1. FROM AN EASY POSE (P.39) WiTH LEFT HEEL CLOSE TO GROIN... KEEP BACK ERECT AND <u>HiPS</u>, <u>LEGS</u>, <u>ANKLES</u>, <u>FEET</u> DEEPLY <u>RELAXED</u>...

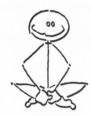

2. HOLD FRONT OF RIGHT <u>ANKLE</u> WITH BOTH HANDS... (LEFT HEEL REMAINS IN PLACE NEAR GROIN)...

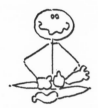

3. BEND ELBOWS TO SLOWLY LiFT RIGHT FOOT AND PULL HEEL TOWARD NAVEL...KEEP SHOULDERS DOWN AND LEVEL...

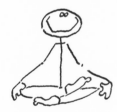

4. LAY OUTER FOOT AND ANKLE (NOT JUST TOES) ACROSS UPPER LEFT THIGH (AS CLOSE TO ABDOMEN AS POSSIBLE)...

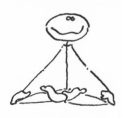

5. HOLD FRONT OF <u>LEFT</u> ANKLE WITH BOTH HANDS...CAREFULLY, SLiDE LEFT FOOT UP OVER RIGHT SHIN...LAY OUTER ANKLE/FOOT ACROSS RIGHT THIGH (BOTH HEELS SHOULD NOW BE CLOSE TO GROIN).. KEEP LOWER BODY AND LEGS DEEPLY RELAXED...FOCUS STRAIGHT AHEAD... [HOLD]...

6. SLiDE LEFT FOOT, THEN RIGHT, TO FLOOR... REPEAT POSE (OTHER SiDE)...REST iN A SEATED POSE.

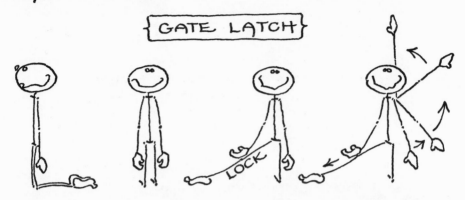

GATE LATCH

1. FROM A KNEELING POSE (P. 40)...EXTEND RIGHT LEG OUT SIDEWAYS, PLACING RIGHT HEEL EXACTLY IN LINE WITH LEFT KNEE...KEEP LEFT THIGH PERPENDICULAR TO FLOOR...LOCK RIGHT KNEE (<u>KEEP RIGHT LEG TIGHTLY LOCKED</u> AND <u>KNEECAP TURNED UP</u> DURING ENTIRE POSE)... LAY BACK OF RIGHT HAND ON RIGHT THIGH...

2. STRETCH LEFT ARM OUT SIDEWAYS AND UP OVER HEAD...REACH GENTLY TOWARD CEILING...

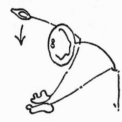

3. <u>KEEP BOTH SHOULDERS AND BOTH HIPBONES EXACTLY SAME DISTANCE FROM FRONT WALL</u>... SLIDE RIGHT HAND DOWN RIGHT LEG AS FAR AS POSSIBLE (WITH LEFT ARM CLOSE TO LEFT EAR)... RELAX NECK AND LAY EAR ON SHOULDER...

4. STRETCH BOTH ARMS AND JOIN PALMS ON FOOT (FACE REMAINS FRAMED <u>BETWEEN</u> ARMS)... FOCUS STRAIGHT AHEAD... HOLD .. (KEEP LEFT ARM EXACTLY OVER EAR)...

5. ROLL UP SLOWLY, REACHING FOR CEILING WITH LEFT ARM AND SLIDING RIGHT HAND UP LEG... RETURN TO A KNEELING POSE...REPEAT POSE, (OTHER SIDE), EXTENDING LEFT LEG.

## { SLEEPING WARRIOR }

1. FROM A THUNDERBOLT POSE (P. 40) SEPARATE FEET JUST ENOUGH TO BE ABLE TO SIT FIRMLY ON FLOOR BETWEEN HEELS...KEEP INNER EDGES OF FEET CLOSE TO HIPS...

(DO NOT CONTINUE IF HIPS OR KNEES LIFT OFF FLOOR)

2. KNEES MUST STAY TOGETHER AND ON FLOOR DURING ENTIRE POSE... LEAN BACKWARD AND BRACE 1 ELBOW AT A TIME ON FLOOR BEHIND HIPS... IF KNEES ARE STILL TOGETHER AND DOWN —

3. LOWER 1 SHOULDER-BLADE AT A TIME TO FLOOR...

4. INTERLOCK FINGERS IN FRONT OF CHEST...CHECK TO BE CERTAIN THAT KNEES, BUTTOCKS, SHOULDER-BLADES AND HEAD ARE ON FLOOR... (LOWER SPINE WILL ARCH SLIGHTLY OFF FLOOR)...

5. STRETCH HANDS TOWARD CEILING, THEN TO FLOOR OVER HEAD...KEEP ARMS STRAIGHT AND NECK SOFT... FOCUS STRAIGHT UP... [HOLD]...

6. UNLOCK FINGERS, SLIDE ARMS DOWN TO SIDES... HOLD OUTER ANKLES... PRESS ELBOWS TO FLOOR...LEAN ON RIGHT ELBOW AND ROLL UP IN 1 SMOOTH MOVEMENT...REST IN A SEATED POSE (P. 38 ).

## { SHOULDER STAND }

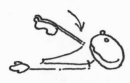

1. FROM A SUPINE POSE (P. 40) KEEP ARMS CLOSE TO BODY... BEND LEGS...DRAW KNEES TO CHEST...KEEP LEGS TOGETHER...

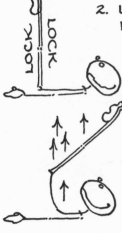

2. UNFOLD LEGS STRAIGHT UP...LOCK KNEES... STRETCH SHOULDERS DOWN, AWAY FROM NECK... STAY IN THIS POSITION AT LEAST 30 SECONDS...

3. GENTLY PRESS FULL LENGTH OF ARMS AGAINST FLOOR TO RAISE HIPS OFF FLOOR AND PUSH FEET TOWARD CEILING...

4. BEND ELBOWS AND BRACE PALMS AGAINST SACRUM...KEEP ELBOWS SHOULDER-WIDTH APART...

5. SLOWLY WALK HANDS UP SPINE TOWARD HEAD TO GRADUALLY STRAIGHTEN LEGS AND BODY...

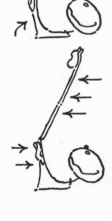

6. CREATE 1 STRAIGHT LINE FROM 7TH VERTEBRA ⟶ HEELS...RELAX FEET...STRETCH BACKS OF THIGHS TOWARD CEILING...TIGHTEN BUTTOCKS...<u>RELAX</u> <u>FACE</u>, <u>THROAT</u>, <u>NECK</u> AND <u>SHOULDERS</u>...BALANCE ON <u>SOFT</u> SHOULDERS AND NECK... FOCUS STRAIGHT UP... HOLD ...

7. BEND AND LOWER KNEES TO FACE (SHINS VERTICAL)...EXTEND ARMS AGAIN...LAY FEET BACK OVER HEAD AND ROLL SPINE DOWN 1 VERTEBRA AT A TIME (KNEES BENT, THIGHS CLOSE TO CHEST, FEET OVER FACE, NECK SOFT)... REST IN A SUPINE POSE.

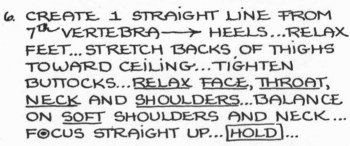

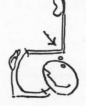

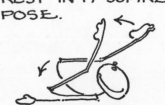

## { SLEEPING FROG }

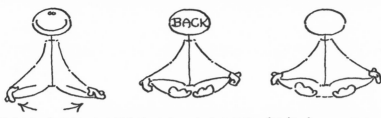

1 FROM A THUNDERBOLT POSE (P. 40) SPREAD KNEES AS FAR APART AS POSSIBLE...

2 SEPARATE TIPS OF BIG TOES JUST ENOUGH TO ALLOW HIPS TO REST FIRMLY ON FLOOR INSIDE OF FEET... (INNER CURVE OF FOOT SHOULD LIE CLOSE TO OUTER CURVE OF HIP)...<u>RELAX FEET</u>, <u>ANKLES</u>, <u>KNEES</u> AND ALLOW <u>GRAVITY</u> TO LOWER HIPS TO FLOOR...

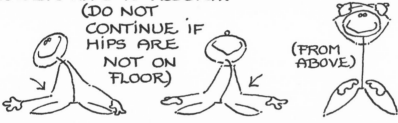

(DO NOT CONTINUE IF HIPS ARE NOT ON FLOOR)

(FROM ABOVE)

3 SLOWLY LEAN BACKWARD AND PLACE 1 ELBOW AT A TIME ON FLOOR... IF THERE IS STILL RESERVE STRETCH IN KNEES AND THIGHS, LOWER 1 SHOULDERBLADE AT A TIME ON FLOOR...FOLD FOREARMS OVER HEAD...RELAX ENTIRE BODY...FOCUS STRAIGHT UP... HOLD ...

4. BRACE ELBOWS ON FLOOR NEAR WAIST... ROLL OVER-AND-UP SLOWLY (TAKING WEIGHT ON 1 ELBOW AND PRESSING OTHER HAND AGAINST FLOOR)... CENTER KNEES...REST IN A THUNDERBOLT POSE.

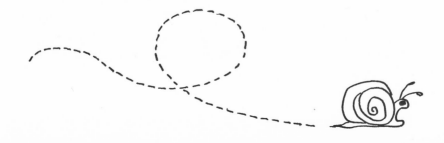

{ FULL MOON }

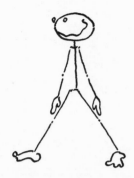

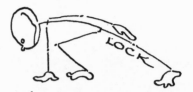

1. FROM AN ANGLED FOOT POSE (P. 41 TOES TURNED RIGHT, FEET 2½ FEET APART)... TURN UPPER BODY RIGHT (STERNUM IN LINE WITH FOOT)... LAY RIGHT PALM ON FRONT OF RIGHT THIGH, LEFT PALM ON BACK OF LEFT THIGH... (LEFT ARM REMAINS STRAIGHT WITH LEFT HAND REACHING TOWARD LEFT HEEL)...

2. IN 1 FLUID MOVEMENT: BEND RIGHT KNEE, SLIDE RIGHT PALM DOWN THIGH/OFF KNEE, LEAN FORWARD OVER BENT LEG, PLACE RIGHT HAND ON FLOOR ABOUT 10 INCHES IN FRONT OF RIGHT FOOT.. PLACE RIGHT THUMB IN LINE WITH OUTER RIGHT HIP... LOCK LEFT KNEE..

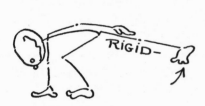

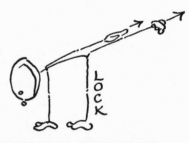

3. SLOWLY STRAIGHTEN AND LOCK RIGHT KNEE WHILE LIFTING LEFT FOOT OFF FLOOR... FOCUS ON FLOOR... DO NOT LEAN ON RIGHT HAND...

4. STRETCH LEFT HEEL AWAY FROM BODY.. TURN LEFT KNEECAP TOWARD FRONT WALL... HOLD LEFT LEG AS HIGH AS POSSIBLE... [HOLD]...

5. SLOWLY BEND RIGHT KNEE AGAIN TO LOWER RIGID LEFT LEG (LEFT FOOT SHOULD RETURN TO ITS ORIGINAL POSITION ON FLOOR).. SLIDE RIGHT HAND UP LEG AND LOCK RIGHT KNEE... TURN TOES AND BODY FORWARD.. REPEAT POSE (OTHER SIDE)... REST IN A STANDING POSE (P. 38 ).

## {POSE OF KNOWLEDGE}

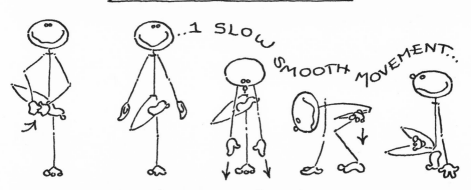

...1 SLOW SMOOTH MOVEMENT...

1. FROM A STANDING POSE (P. 38) SEPARATE FEET 1 INCH... BEND AND RAISE RIGHT KNEE... HOLD FRONT OF RIGHT <u>ANKLE</u> WITH BOTH HANDS...PLACE OUTER EDGE OF FOOT-ANKLE ACROSS FRONT OF LEFT THIGH (CLOSE TO HIP)...

2. GENTLY PRESS RIGHT KNEE DOWN AND BACK...

3. FOCUS ON FLOOR NEAR TOES...LEAN DOWN, REACHING FOR FLOOR

4. BEND STANDING LEG AND SMOOTHLY LOWER BODY INTO A FULL SQUAT (ALLOWING RIGHT HEEL TO LIFT OFF FLOOR NATURALLY)...TOUCH FINGERTIPS TO FLOOR FOR BALANCE...

5. SIT BACK ON RIGHT HEEL, CENTERING HEEL BETWEEN BUTTOCKS...MOVE HANDS CAREFULLY BACKWARD (1 AT A TIME) TO TOUCH FINGERS ON FLOOR <u>NEAR OUTER HIPS</u>... SIT UP STRAIGHT...RELAX RIGHT LEG AND SHOULDERS... GENTLY LIFT STERNUM...FOCUS STRAIGHT AHEAD...

6. BALANCE ON LEFT FOOT... ⟵FOCUS— JOIN PALMS IN FRONT OF CHEST... [HOLD]...

7. TOUCH FLOOR AGAIN NEAR HIPS... SLIDE RIGHT FOOT OFF LEFT KNEE...BRING FEET TOGETHER... STAND UP SLOWLY...REPEAT POSE ON OTHER SIDE... ,BALANCING ON RIGHT FOOT...REST IN A STANDING POSE.

SALUTATION TO THE

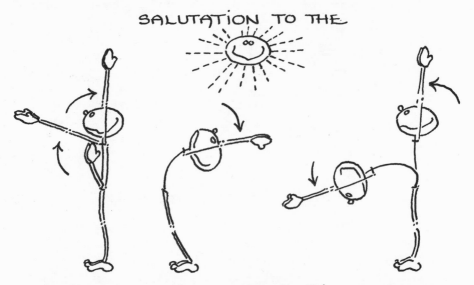

1. FROM A STANDING POSE (P. 38) SEPARATE PARALLEL FEET 1 INCH... JOIN PALMS IN FRONT OF CHEST... STRETCH ARMS FORWARD AND UP OVER HEAD...
2. <u>UNLOCK</u> <u>KNEES</u>...TIGHTEN BUTTOCK MUSCLES...PUSH HIPS FORWARD... ARCH BACK AND STRETCH ARMS GENTLY BACK (EARS TOUCHING UPPER ARMS)...
3. REACH TOWARD CEILING... LOCK KNEES... STRETCH FORWARD AND DOWN...

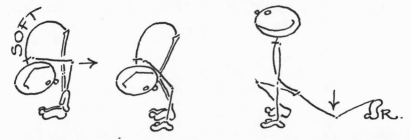

4. HOLD ACHILLES TENDON OR BACK OF HEEL WITH EACH HAND...RELAX NECK, ABDOMEN, SHOULDERS...BEND ELBOWS BACKWARD TO PULL CHEST TO THIGHS...
5. PLACE PALMS ON FLOOR NEAR OUTER EDGES OF FEET...(BEND KNEES IF NECESSARY)...
6. EXTEND RIGHT LEG BACKWARD (IN LINE WITH HIP)...REST ON TOES AND KNEE... KEEP LEFT FOOT FLAT ON FLOOR...

## SALUTATION TO THE

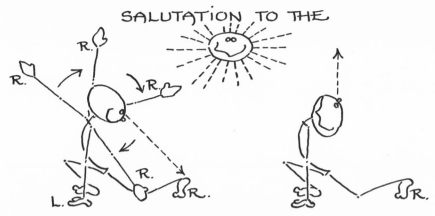

7. STRETCH RIGHT ARM FORWARD, UP OVER HEAD AND BACK TO HOLD INNER RIGHT KNEE...PRESS AGAINST KNEE...LOOK OVER RIGHT SHOULDER AND FOCUS ON RIGHT HEEL...

8. TURN CHEST FORWARD AND DROP RIGHT HAND TO ORIGINAL PLACE ON FLOOR... RELAX NECK AND FOCUS ON CEILING...

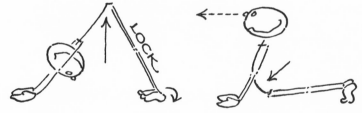

9. STRETCH LEFT LEG BACK (FEET TOGETHER)...LOCK KNEES AND ELBOWS... RAISE HIPS AS HIGH AS POSSIBLE...RELAX NECK...PRESS HEELS TO FLOOR...

10. WITH ELBOWS AND KNEES <u>LOCKED</u>, GLIDE FORWARD TO LOWER HIPS...BALANCE ON PALMS AND TOES...(KEEP SHOULDERS DOWN AND NECK LONG)...

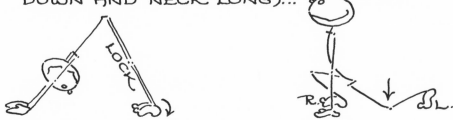

11. RAISE HIPS AGAIN INTO POSITION 9...

12. SLIDE RIGHT FOOT FORWARD BETWEEN HANDS...KEEP LEFT KNEE ON FLOOR...

SALUTATION TO THE

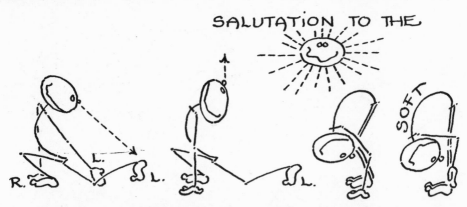

13. STRETCH LEFT ARM FORWARD, UP OVER
    HEAD AND BACK TO HOLD INNER LEFT
    KNEE... FOCUS ON LEFT HEEL...
14. TURN CHEST FORWARD AND DROP LEFT
    HAND TO ORIGINAL POSITION ON FLOOR...
    RELAX NECK... FOCUS ON CEILING...
15. SLIDE LEFT FOOT FORWARD BETWEEN
    HANDS... STRAIGHTEN LEGS...
16. HOLD BACK OF EACH HEEL... RELAX
    ABDOMEN AND UPPER BODY... BEND
    ELBOWS BACKWARD TO PULL CHEST TO
    THIGHS...

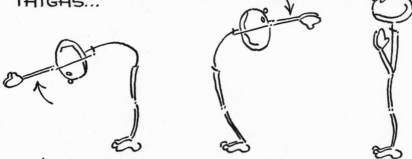

17. JOIN PALMS... STRETCH ARMS FORWARD
    AND UP OVER HEAD...
18. UNLOCK KNEES... TIGHTEN BUTTOCK
    MUSCLES... PUSH HIPS FORWARD... ARCH
    BACK AND STRETCH ARMS GENTLY
    BACKWARD (EARS BETWEEN ARMS)...
19. STRETCH ARMS UP TOWARD CEILING,
    THEN FORWARD... CENTER PALMS IN
    FRONT OF STERNUM... BEGIN AGAIN.

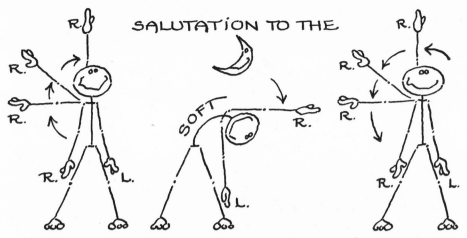

SALUTATION TO THE

1. SEPARATE FEET 3 FEET APART IN A SPREAD FOOT POSE (P. 39)...STRETCH RIGHT ARM OUT SIDEWAYS AND UP OVER HEAD...
2. SLIDE LEFT HAND DOWN LEFT LEG...STRETCH RIGHT ARM OVER EAR (LEVEL WITH FLOOR) ...RELAX NECK...DO NOT TWIST SPINE...
3. ROLL UP SLOWLY TO STRAIGHTEN BACK.... FLOAT ARM DOWN TO SIDE...

   [REPEAT STEPS 1, 2, 3 ON OTHER SIDE]...

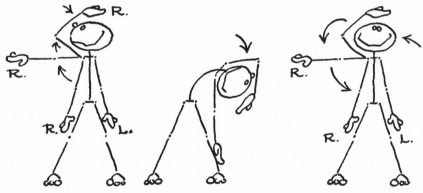

4. STRETCH RIGHT ARM OUT SIDEWAYS AND UP OVER HEAD...BEND RIGHT ELBOW...FLOAT RIGHT PALM OVER HEAD...TURN FACE INTO INNER RIGHT ELBOW...
5. SLIDE LEFT PALM DOWN OUTER LEFT LEG...
6. STRAIGHTEN UP SLOWLY...EXTEND RIGHT ARM OUT SIDEWAYS...FLOAT HAND DOWN TO OUTER THIGH...FACE FORWARD...

   [REPEAT STEPS 4, 5, 6 ON OTHER SIDE]...

SALUTATION TO THE

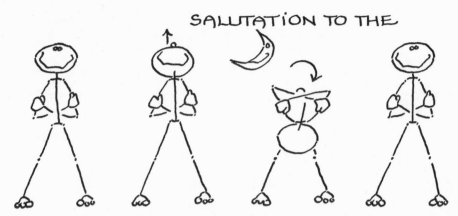

7. FOLD ARMS BEHIND BACK...HOLD ELBOWS...
8. ARCH SPINE BACKWARD...RELAX NECK AND FOCUS ON CEILING...
9. ROLL BODY FORWARD AND DOWN... RELAX NECK...
10. ROLL UP SLOWLY UNTIL BACK IS ERECT...

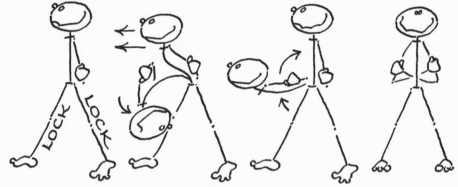

11. TURN TOES AND BODY RIGHT IN AN ANGLED FOOT POSE (P. 41)... LOCK KNEES...
12. STRETCH CHIN OUT AND DOWN OVER RIGHT SHIN...RELAX NECK...
13. ROLL UP SLOWLY TO STRAIGHTEN BACK...
14. TURN TOES AND BODY FORWARD...

    [REPEAT STEPS 11-14, TURNING LEFT]...

15. RELEASE ELBOWS...LOWER ARMS TO SIDES AND BEGIN AGAIN.

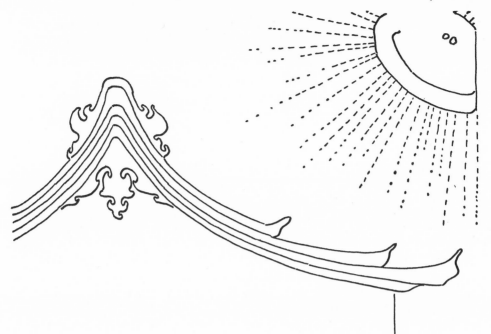

DEDICATED TO~
MY FAMILY, MY STUDENTS,
AND TO MOTHER NATURE
(THANK YOU FOR HELPING
ME CHASE MY DRAGONS).

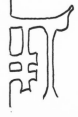